Highly Sensitive Person

Stop Emotional Overload with Eq Strategies

(Stop Anxiety and Negative Energy in Highly Sensitive Person)

Jeremy Rogers

Published By **Bella Frost**

Jeremy Rogers

All Rights Reserved

Highly Sensitive Person: Stop Emotional Overload with Eq Strategies (Stop Anxiety and Negative Energy in Highly Sensitive Person)

ISBN 978-1-998927-45-6

Legal & Disclaimer

The information contained in this book is not designed to replace or take the place of any form of medicine or professional medical advice. The information in this book has been provided for educational & entertainment purposes only.

The information contained in this book has been compiled from sources deemed reliable, and it is accurate to the best of the Author's knowledge; however, the Author cannot guarantee its accuracy and validity and cannot be held liable for any errors or omissions. Changes are periodically made to this book. You must consult your doctor or get professional medical advice before using any of the suggested remedies, techniques, or information in this book.

Table Of Contents

Chapter 1: What exactly is an "HSP" (Highly Sensitive People)?

The term "highly sensitive person" refers to someone with heightened or deeper central nervous systems sensitivity to emotional, social, and physical stimuli.

This can be referred to as having sensory processing sensitivity (or SPS) by some people.

Although "too sensitive", a negative term that describes overly sensitive people is used a lot, this personality characteristic has its advantages and disadvantages.

Elaine Aron was a psychologist and Arthur Aron was the first to use the phrase "very sensitive individual" during the 1990s. Interest in the idea has grown ever since Elaine Aron's 1996 book, "The Highly Sensitive People", was published.

How can you tell whether you are an HPS?

Ever been told that you were "too sensitive" or "shouldn't be thinking so much" by someone? If they're coming from someone you find too insensitive, or who needs to think a bit more, this is especially true. HSP (highly sensitive person) could be one of these.

It is important to remember that HSP doesn't mean you have a mental illness. There is no official diagnosis for high-sensitive people. High sensitivity can be described as being more open to both positive and adverse effects.

There are several types of high sensitivity.

Researchers who identified this personality feature believe that HSPs share many of the same characteristics and qualities as other people.

Avoid watching violent movies or TV because it can be too intense and cause you to feel uneasy

The ability to be deeply touched by beauty, regardless of whether it is found in nature, art or the human spirit.

Arons' complex inner life is rich in deep ideas and powerful emotions. This helps people to identify themselves as HSPs. They also developed a personality assessment, or highly sensitive person test. Aron's Highly Sensitive Persons Scale was its name (HSPS).

How pervasive are HSPs

Around 20% of the population are highly sensitive.

The majority of sensitive people are not common. Society tends to revolve around those who take things less seriously and pay more attention.

For highly sensitive individuals, it may be helpful to find techniques for handling the pressures they sometimes experience. This is true both for people who know their sensitive levels and those who have loved ones who show higher levels.

Why are people sensitive to high levels?

It is possible that highly sensitive people are highly sensitive for many reasons, including their environment, genetics, genes, early experiences, and evolution.

High sensitivity is not only a characteristic of humans but also 100 other species. Research shows that high sensitivity might have evolved to be a survival advantage as HSPs are always on the lookout for potential predators or potentially hazardous circumstances. Worry is often a result of being constantly alert, even when there are no imminent threats.

Study after study suggests that high levels of sensitivity can be triggered by a lack in parental love and affection during childhood. Negative early experiences are also a factor. As a youngster, you could be more likely to become an HSP.

Genetics can influence high sensitivity. The dopamine receptor could be involved. It can impact personality and cause some people to be more sensitive than others. Also, high levels of sensitivity are often inherited.

If you are sensitive in your family, there is a higher chance that you will develop it.

A person's genetic makeup could be affected by early life events that are not favorable, which can increase their chance of developing HSP.

Similar traits and conditions

Sensitivity can sometimes be confused with other personality qualities and mental health issues.

Introversion is when introverts are subject to excessive stimuli. Introverts are particularly sensitive to stimuli like large groups or parties. HSPs can be sensitive to noise and light, but they might also feel overwhelmed by social cues.

SPD, disorder of sensory Processing: SPD-afflicted people and very sensitive people might be resistant to sensory input. HSPs may not have motor impairments, but SPD could. SPD might cause under reactivity. HSPs can also overreact towards sensory inputs.

Autism does have high sensitivity. HSPs are often overloaded with sensory information, but autism sufferers may be hypersensitive (or hypersensitive) to it.

Attention-deficit/hyperactivity disorder (ADHD): HSPs may potentially be mistakenly diagnosed with ADHD (ADHD). ADHD patients and HSPs are both hypersensitive to stimuli. But HSPs can also be diagnosed with ADHD. ADHD sufferers may have cognitive symptoms like trouble concentrating, paying attention, or difficulty paying attention.

While high sensitivity can be misdiagnosed as other mental health conditions, it is important for people to understand that high sensitive may also be associated with other mental illness disorders. It is possible to have ADHD or SPD while simultaneously being an HSP.

Effects of the HSP Status

Being an HSP comes with its own set of benefits and drawbacks. It is easy to take offense when people are trying to help or be kind. It is easy for people to react violently to daily tensions or problems in relationships.

An HSP doesn't automatically mean you are a bad person. They are more easily perceived. It is possible to be more negatively affected than others.

A variety of factors can influence your life as an HSP, such as:

You can avoid being overwhelmed by circumstances. Certain situations, such as tension, aggression and conflict, may have a greater impact on sensitive people. This could make them more likely to avoid undesirable situations.

Passion or beauty can cause you to feel profoundly moved. People with high levels are more sensitive than others and have stronger emotional reactions to beauty. They often weep after watching touching videos.

You may be very close with certain people. Friendships with HSPs are vital and can often lead to lasting relationships. Being a friend or family member who is sensitive and compassionate is a great asset.

You might be grateful for your life. People with high levels of sensitive senses may find it difficult to appreciate things like a good wine or a great meal. While they might experience more existential grief, they might also feel more thankfulness for what is available to them in life.

There are many benefits to being an HSP, including the ability for empathy. Empathy is a skill that can help you have healthy relationships and live an emotionally rich lifestyle. It's essential to differentiate between your feelings and those of others.

Although HSPs have lower lows than other people, they have the potential for higher highs.

You can be an HSP and have more strength and less struggle if you learn how to handle it. You can do this to understand yourself and others who are sensitive.

How to make a Stress Reduction plan that works.

It is not surprising that highly sensitive people experience greater stress when faced with difficult circumstances. Worrying about other people may cause them to be more sensitive.

Social stress is considered more exhausting than any other type of stress by most people. This can be especially true for those who see many possible outcomes in a confrontation and can sense tension or animosity when others cannot.

The following are sensitive and particular factors that could cause extreme stress:

Busy schedules

Some people enjoy the rush of being busy, but not all. HPSs, on the other hand, can experience anxiety and stress when there is too much work to do. It can be stressful to deal with the pressure of these situations and to keep in mind the uncertainty of not being able complete all the work.

Requirements of others

People with high levels in sensitivity are more sensitive than others and can be aware of the needs, emotions, and desires of others. They dislike disappointing others. HSPs may find it hard to say no.

Highly sensitive people often have the hardest critics: themselves. They are usually resentful of other people's pleasures or, at the very minimum, they are aware of them when there are negative feelings.

Conflicts

HSPs could be more stressed out by conflict. Even if they don't say anything wrong, HSPs could be more aware that problems are developing in their relationships. In some cases, people may mistakenly interpret signals as being signs of anger or conflict.

Comparing social

Social comparisons may make people who are very sensitive more susceptible to pressure. They may experience their own emotions more strongly than the negative feelings of another person.

Potentially positive outcomes can give way to more bad ones when the disagreement becomes worse. They could be more aware that there is potential for improvement, and they might not be as unhappy.

They may feel even worse when they realize a relationship is ending.

People with high levels of sensitiveness may be more affected by the end a relationship and might ruminate more.

Tolerations

These regular energy drains are called tolerations by Life Coaches. It's things we tolerate that aren't necessary but can cause stress. Bad odors can be perceived more strongly and make it harder for HSPs to relax. Distractions can also seem more stressful to HSPs who are trying to focus.

People with high sensitivity to the environment are more likely be surprised. People with high sensitivity can become "hungry" when they are hungry. They don't have the energy to deal with it. In this way, highly sensitive people can become more sensitive due to everyday stresses.

Personal setbacks

HSPs are more susceptible to self-doubt as they are the hardest judges of themselves. A humiliating mistake could be something they remember for a while, and they might feel worse than a normal person about it.

They are not happy to be judged or observed while they're working on difficult tasks. Although they are often perfectionists, they may be more aware of how stress can impact them and what they can do to reduce it.

The Influence of Personality On Physical and Mental Health

How to manage Stress as a High-Stress Person

Learn coping skills if your personality is more sensitive. You may need to protect yourself from stimuli that are too stimulating if you're sensitive. A wall should be built between you, excessive sensory stimulation, and your body. Recognize your stressors, and learn how to avoid them.

Planning pleasant activities will help you to avoid future stress.

Avoid stress-inducing activity and people like horror movies. These can drain your positive energies, set high expectations, or make you feel self conscious.

Establish a boundary in life and learn how to say "no" to requests that are too difficult.

You should create a secure space. Make your home a peaceful haven.

Empathy is a higher quality than empathy and you will experience stronger emotions, no matter how favorable or negative. Lows are not always easy, but they can bring you opportunities to improve your stress levels and relationships. To avoid getting overwhelmed in stressful situations, you need to plan how you will manage your emotions.

Chapter 2: How to increase your emotional intelligence and manage emotional exhaustion.

A person may experience emotional weariness after experiencing extreme stress in their professional and personal lives.

People feeling emotionally exhausted can feel overburdened, exhausted and depleted. Even though individuals may not be able to see the warning signs immediately, these feelings often persist over a prolonged period.

This may have a profound impact on one's day, relationships, and behavior. This article examines emotional tiredness, its causes, and potential risk factors. It also discusses some of the treatments and techniques available to combat it.

What causes emotional fatigue

You may feel tired or depressed due to persistent stress.

Most often, emotional weariness occurs after a stressful experience.

There are many factors that can lead to emotional weariness depending on one's tolerance of stress and the circumstances surrounding them at the moment.

The following could cause emotional exhaustion.

Going through major life events, such a divorce or loss of a family member, being a caregiver due to financial hardship, having children or having a baby, being homeless, trying to balance several responsibilities like job, family and education, or working long hours within a stressful environment.

People often feel exhausted by their lives. They might feel powerless over their lives. Or they may not be managing life's obligations and taking care of themselves.

Emotions serve to incite us and provide internal cues which aid in understanding or making decisions (such as a gut feeling).

Accessing key signals is the key to preventing emotional contagion.

Social Cooperation and Bonding

Emotions also aid in building relationships with others and allowing them to work together. They are also a social signaling tool. Understanding and responding to other people's emotions can be crucial to social communication. It plays a vital role in interpersonal interactions.

It allows us to communicate clearly and builds stronger, more meaningful connections with our families, friends, and loved ones. It allows us to understand and give clues to others through our interactions. These signals may include the physical expressions of emotion such as facial expressions that are related to the emotions we feel.

One example is that there are 90 muscles in our faces. Only 30 are used for emotion. This knowledge can help us to make informed decisions on how to interact.

Some feelings can be pleasant, while some may be uncomfortable. This does not necessarily mean that certain emotions are more positive than others. To avoid spreading "sad," it is important not to pretend to be "glad." It's all about being able recognize the messages that each emotion is trying convey to you.

A higher emotional quotient

Emotional intelligence (EI), or increasing our emotional intelligence, is the first step towards understanding how to use emotional contagion as an effective tool to improve your life. John Salavoy and John Mayer were two social psychologists who first proposed the idea for EI in 1990. Emotional intelligence can be described as the ability to recognize, express, and manage one's own emotions and those of others.

Emotions are vital to our survival. We all have emotions to motivate us, protect us against danger, and increase our pleasure. Why does emotion have such a negative reputation?

Why emotions are misunderstood

All of us were taught from an early age how to express ourselves. Many of us were caught in an ironic situation.

We can learn from our ancestors how to suppress our emotions. Many of us might have heard advice such "Don't weep," or "There's no reason for you to feel unhappy." Drama queens are girls who openly express their emotions. Girls who freely expressed their feelings might have been called sissies.

Of all the motivations for offering such counsel, comforting or mentoring a young person is often the most effective. The cultural message was that we should suppress our emotions or at minimum keep them hidden from others to satisfy ourselves.

The problem is when we become so good at suppressing and expressing emotions that we lose sight of the important purposes they serve. Negative emotions can have valuable functions. Emotions are like a phone ringing. It is trying to relay a key message. They can be used to indicate the areas of our life that need attention.

Denying your feelings can hinder you from being able to connect with yourself. Realizing your need to listen to their messages is the first step.

EI can still be developed and enhanced with practice. Follow these seven tips to improve your emotional intelligence.

Build your first somatic vocabulary

Develop the ability feel your emotions through physical sensations. Emotional intelligence (EI), can be expressed verbally or through a somatic language. The following example illustrates how emotions can be embodied. Even though you may know the causes of your anger but not the feeling,

It's possible to feel this when you're feeling upset

Your brow wrinkles

Your pupils feel constrained

Your jaw is extended outward.

You have pursed the lips.

Your body is racing.

The sensation of a rapid increase in breath speed is felt

You're clenching fists.

Your body is prepping for battle. This tells you that you are furious and lets others know.

2. Give yourself space to express your emotions

Without passing judgement, reflect on your emotions. Emotions do not have to be wrong or right, good or bad. They can help you develop self-awareness by providing knowledge. You should sit down at least twice daily to assess your health and well-being.

It might take some time before the emotions surface. Enjoy a few moments of quiet. Recognize the emotions you feel, where they are felt in your body and give them a name. Naming an emotion is a useful technique for decreasing its intensity or increasing its positive impact.

Pay attention how your emotions influence, distract from, accentuate, or challenge. EI is built around self-awareness.

3. Listen to others' feelings

Open-mindedness and an effort to understand others' feelings is important. Be open-minded and recognize that every situation can be viewed from multiple angles. Try to understand the motives behind someone's different emotional responses and how they view it. Listen to and watch radio and TV conversations. Look at the arguments from all sides. Search for any nuanced issues that need further investigation. Challenge your beliefs.

4. Be aware of the impact your actions have on others.

Take the time to evaluate your impact on others and listen to their points of view. You should be open to criticism. It is possible to be seen differently by other people than you are yourself. This is not about wrong or right. It is useful to reflect on how perceptions may differ and the potential effects of such differences.

Tell someone you trust about your emotional reactions. Even if it isn't what you agree with, taking the time to listen to their thoughts can help you avoid mistakes and see if your actions have the desired effects.

5. You should be aware of your emotions

Look at the relationship between your emotions & conduct. Consider how you react to a certain emotion. Are you angry when you feel overwhelmed? Do you become anxious and lose sight on what you were doing when overwhelmed? Do you withdraw from or disconnect when you are feeling embarrassed or insecure

6. Reputation is key to your success

Accept responsibility for your thoughts and actions. Only you can control your emotions and actions. Your thoughts, your behavior and how you react are all up to you.

7. Emotional Integrity

Learn how you can control your emotions. This is possible only if your emotions are conscious. Empathic transparency and openness are key to allowing others to read you.

You should tell people when it is happy and when it is sad. Develop a strategy for managing your emotions to avoid harming others.

Listen when people are expressing their emotions.

Instead of reacting and rushing, try responding instead. You can use "the pause" to respond. Instead of responding out of emotion, pause to gather facts and then reply after considering it.

Take a deep breath. Stress or a bad day could affect your ability control emotions. Emotions impact our physiological functions. Stress can make us feel like danger is around. If you feel stressed, just take a moment to calm down and relax. This will likely open your heart and mind, which will make it easier to build positive relationships with others.

You can improve your emotional intelligence (EI), however, it takes some time. It is an ongoing process. Also, you cannot manage your emotions perfectly. Remember to keep the motto "Progress is not perfection" in your mind.

These guidelines are easy to follow.

Give yourself a highfive. You're getting closer to using the power and influence of emotional contagion for your benefit, rather than against.

Chapter 3: How to identify toxic relationships and avoid falling in Love too soon in order to maintain a strong relationship.

Did you ever wonder if your love is too quick? You're not alone if this is you. Frank Sinatra's "I Fall In Love Too Easily", a song that was later covered by Chet Baker, is a true masterpiece. Its words, especially lines such as the following, have made Frank Sinatra's song a popular choice for many people.

Although I have been duped in my past, my heart needs to be educated. Yet, I continue to fall in love with too fast and so easily.

You might find it easy to fall in love, even if you don't like the song.

If you are a mature single person looking to find a partner for life, then you may be asking yourself how to fall deeply in love. When you are looking for the perfect one for you, you may find yourself falling in love faster than you expected.

Sometimes you may give in too quickly to your emotions only to be disappointed when the other person doesn't feel exactly the same. You might feel passionate emotions and think that you are in a committed relationship. But those emotions can pass quickly. This could lead to an unhappy relationship with your partner.

Most likely, you aren't trying to harm yourself or anyone else with your amorous pursuits. You might be unable to let go of your desire to love someone. It's possible to feel alone. There are many safe and healthy ways you can find love.

Continue reading to learn about falling for love and determine if you are able to answer the question, "Does my love make me fall in love too quickly?" You may find this information relevant.

Don't date

It might be a good idea for you to stop saying, "I miss love", but you know that you cannot see the truth about a relationship because of your emotional state. You are free to take as many breaks as you need until it is easier to focus on what is good for you.

You should not avoid dating if your goal is to find a long-lasting relationship. This is a temporary measure that you can use to help you learn coping skills and build a connection.

You can use this chance to learn more about your self while getting away from the dating world. Go on dates, do errands and be your own judge. Love can only be found when you understand yourself and are open to accepting others.

Even more interesting, research has found that engaging in solitude can help reduce stress and improve your ability to control your emotions.

It could be hard to let go of the inner voice that keeps telling you how you want to love. It is possible to give yourself the space you need to become more mature and emotionally mature if your patience and kindness are shown to yourself.

Take your Time

You have decided to stop dating. You were alone on the balcony and enjoyed mimosas as you reminisce about being single. You might have been dating casually and now feel ready for a committed relationship.

Whatever brought you to this place, you might be eager or afraid to go back to the real you.

It could be tempting for you to begin dating immediately after you have found the right person. You and your partner may have a strong first attraction that makes it seem like there is no stopping you.

Remember all the hard work that you put into getting to this point. Keep in mind all the work you did to build stability inside.

No matter how difficult the first few stages of a relationship can be, it is worth taking the time to enjoy them and not rush to get to the next. By sharing more information about yourself with your spouse, you can make sure that they are on the same page.

You can benefit from being honest with your partner right from the beginning to help you decide if they are the right one. If you take things slow when you first get to know each other, you may discover more about them and decide if it is worth the effort.

A speed race is not the same as a slow, beautiful trip. The same applies to romantic connections. Even though it might be exciting and spectacular, there is always danger. Furthermore, the driver must be highly skilled. The speed race is often as fast as the driver started. If you're trying to build a lasting relationship, slowing down could help you save your time.

Take your steps back

If you find yourself saying "I fall for too easy," as Frank Sinatra sang, it may be time to take a step back. Maybe your past relationships were quite turbulent. You may find yourself confused by situations that quickly go wrong.

You might have experienced similar circumstances before and wondered what went wrong. Sometimes it can be difficult for you to be open with yourself about the things that are preventing you and your partner from finding the love you long for.

You can't just play the same songs over and over and expect them to sound different.

You might find it helpful to step back from the relationship and examine your past relationships. Are there any patterns you can see? Did you get the same answers from several people? Do you often find yourself telling yourself stories from past relationships? Do any recurring defensive mechanisms exist?

Do you think you can change or adjust these things? Are there ways to improve your current situation and help you reach your goals? How you answer these question and how well you know yourself will help you understand how potential partners view you.

It's normal to struggle to maintain relationships, to choose the right partners, or to find fulfillment in your romantic endeavors. It will only help you know yourself better. Ask yourself questions about who and what you want to be in this position.

Try putting yourself out there in situations that are not your usual ones if you feel like you're going in circles. There might be new people at your neighborhood park or community center who could disrupt your routine.

More time spent with friends

If we have a new companion that we are passionate about, it may be easier to overlook our friendships. To make room for this new relationship, you may need to sacrifice your friendship goals because everyone has a busy life.

Friends can be a great way to relax and focus, even if you're not in a relationship. Even though it is tempting to get caught in the excitement of your new boyfriend, having a solid support group of friends can help you long-term. Your pals can be there to support you in your excitement and worries. If you decide that it is time to change, your friends could also help.

It is essential to make sure the important people in your life feel special. Neglecting or ignoring your pals in a relationship can lead to you not receiving the support you need.

This old saying, "Partners may come and go but friends are always there," might be true. There is a greater risk of a relationship ending abruptly than a dependable friendship, since all relationships can become emotionally charged. By scheduling time for your buddies, you will make it easier for yourself to enjoy your hobbies and save money.

Be practical

Timing is everything in love and life. Many people believe that they knew their destiny from the moment they met. But, it is possible for love to take time.

Be aware that these are not the usual romantic stories of "love at first glance". If they leave you feeling confused or helpless, remember that these are usually the most exciting exceptions. Realistic expectations can help you be open to all possibilities and people.

Realistic expectations are about allowing your relationship time to grow at its pace. Reliable expectations will help you avoid acting too quickly on your inspirations, which could cause disruption to the natural flow of your relationship.

You will gain a deeper understanding of the person you are working with and a better understanding of your relationship.

It may be difficult at first to get on the same page and communicate with a new spouse. Their timeline may differ from yours. They might have different long-term and short-term goals. Some people fall for someone very quickly. For others, there are certain criteria that must be met before they commit their hearts to someone.

If you fall in love quicker than you would like, it may be difficult for you to stay in this moment. Your creativity and your ability to love will make you stand out. You don't have to be with a potential partner. It's just as important to get to know yourself.

Sites for dating shouldn't be taken seriously.

It might be worth looking into dating services to help you meet someone new, especially if it seems so long since you have met someone you love. This strategy has worked for some people.

There are certain things that you need to be mindful of when online dating.

Your goals may differ from those of others. Talking to potential dates can help you determine if your heart is in the same place as theirs.

Use of dating websites is not always easy. It is not always easy to find meaningful relationships online. Dating sites may directly impact our self-esteem, as they can teach us to think of people and ourselves as things to be judged at face value.

Safety and wellness are important, as they are with all things. It's important to set reasonable expectations and make sure you feel at home with the person and place you are visiting. This will help you give your best shot when you meet someone online.

Consult a specialist

Talking to a professional in mental health could be beneficial if your self-deprecating statements about falling in love are common. This topic may be discussed with you by a therapist if you're interested in becoming more relaxed with yourself while you wait to find the ideal partner.

Maybe you are looking for something deeper and want someone to listen. You might be unable to see why certain things aren't going your way. You are not required to navigate your way through life alone. You might be able to access virtual counseling today.

A counselor can help you to develop healthy, long-lasting habits and be happy. Research shows that online counseling is often more beneficial than in-person therapy. It can be very enlightening and refocusing, to get advice from a qualified counselor on how to meet your spouse.

Online counseling is a fantastic way for many people to get the treatment that they want on their terms. You have many options to get treatment. These include texting, video chats and phone conversations. This allows you to reach your certified counselor at any time.

You might feel more comfortable going to an in-person program rather than signing up for an online service. The online long-term treatment has the same benefits as the in-person sessions and you can do it from your home.

What are the Characteristics of a Healthy Relationship

Healthy relationships are based on compromise and cooperation from both partners. This includes open communication between partners, honesty, trust, respect, and open communication. There are no power differences. Partner's choices are shared, they can accept each others' freedom and act independently, without fear of repercussions. No one is obligated to leave the other partner if a relationship ends.

What healthy relationships look and feel like

Respect for one's space. Your companion doesn't need to be with you all the time.

Your spouse will encourage you and your friends to take part in the activities that you love.

You can freely share your worries and thoughts with your loved one.

Your partner will not pressurize or pressure you into having sexual relations. You can feel physically secure with them.

Because you respect your needs and emotions, it is possible to compromise and negotiate with your spouse when there are differences or conflicts.

These are the elements that make up a solid connection.

The ability to set boundaries allows you and you partner to be able meet each other's needs in a way both of you can live with.

Even if you disagree, communication allows your spouse and you to express your emotions in such a way that the other person feels at ease, heard, and unjudged.

Building trust takes patience. But it allows couples the freedom to be vulnerable with each other because they know they can rely on the other.

This is the most common way to consent to having sex.

The consent you grant once is not an obligation to continue giving it later; consent may be revoked at all times.

Your safety may be put at risk by trying to impose boundaries, open communications, trust, and other positive behavior in abusive relationships. Be aware that abuse can be all about power and control. A person who is abusive may not want to let go of their authority.

Chapter 4: Being a successful HSP and choosing a career.

Highly sensitive persons (HSPs), however, are born with this level. Their neural system is well-suited for it. This ability to empathize and see the nuances of others is a strength. HSPs are people who are sensitive, caring and creative.

An HSP can feel overwhelmed by the everyday sights, sounds, smells and feelings that may be partially missed by others. It can even make life difficult for them.

It takes a combination of two strategies to find the perfect job for someone sensitive.

Utilize your advantages. Many professions, from the arts to the helping professions, could benefit from your empathy for people, and sensitivity towards subtle indications.

Your sensory needs should be considered. If you're constantly overwhelmed by sensory and emotional stimuli, it's better to have a job that allows you to "take a break" as you need it. Also, avoid jobs that frequently expose you loud noises, demanding schedules or other sensory overload.

Let's explore a few careers that may be especially suitable for someone with high levels of sensitivity.

1. Therapist or counselor

The majority of HSPs can empathize with others and are sensitive to their emotions. They can approach someone non-threateningly by picking up subtle nonverbal signs that allow them access to the person's feelings.

These skills may help you be an effective counsellor, psychotherapist, or psychologist. Personal coaching, which may resemble counseling in some ways, could also be covered under this heading.

Aside from the fact that you usually only work with one client (or a couple) at any given time and have breaks between meetings, these circumstances allow you to better serve your clients' needs.

As you are likely to have some control over the environment you work in, you may create the sights, sounds, and textures that are relaxing and pleasing to you. This is important for HSPs.

Remote counseling sessions are becoming increasingly popular, making it possible for HSP counselors create an environment that is welcoming and supportive.

2. Professor in University

A majority of college instructors are only able to teach for an hour at a stretch, with breaks, in contrast to elementary teachers, who may have to "perform for hours".

The arrangement works in the same way as therapy but provides the HSPs with the peace and quiet they need. Additionally, you have more control over the atmosphere, pace, and classroom type.

Another advantage is the ability to work with people who have an interest and are willing to go, and to share your knowledge and enthusiasm about a topic with others.

3. A creator/artist

People who are exceptionally sensitive may be able to become great artists due to how deeply they feel connected into the sensory world. They have an innate aesthetic sense, and can communicate their ideas to others through their creative endeavours.

Your sensibility may be a valuable asset, no matter what medium you choose to express it via creative production.

Creativity is an excellent way to be creative and to establish a comfortable pace.

4. A health professional

Do you see a pattern here? You can make a difference by using your unique talents and creating a loving environment.

To meet the medical needs of your customers, you might be most successful if you focus on holistic health such as chiropractic, acupuncture, herbal medicines, or massage therapy.

It depends on the situation, you could even succeed as an obstetrician or traditional practitioner. If you are a private practitioner, you can use your skills to create a successful practice. Working as a physician or nurse in an ER is not the best option.

5. Author, songwriter, or editor?

The literary and editorial arts give you the opportunity to use your creative sense and calm attention towards detail to your advantage.

This kind of job is often done in sensitive settings, and can sometimes be done at your own office.

It does matter what kind of work and how fast it is done. You may avoid working in noisy, fast-paced newsrooms that are loud and difficult to read.

Focusing on creative and serious tasks from home or in a less noisy environment would be a better choice.

5. Museum/Library Curator

It is a great place to share your love of literature, history and art.

You might split your time working in the background with interacting in a low-key setting. You'll have the ability to harness your unique talents and engage others, while also working solo, which can give you some much-needed solitude, peace, and meditation.

Another quality that makes a sensitive person highly sensitive is their desire for beauty in the world. Literature and art may help them to achieve this.

7. Any freelance work

One drawback to self-employment is the need to market yourself and often get turned away. These might be problematic for HSPs because of their sensitive nature.

Calling or attending meetings in person can be stressful. Therefore, one way to reduce stress is to do your online marketing. A mix of part time jobs and freelancing can be a great way to expand your clientele.

If you are well-known, you can leverage your reputation to do a lot more networking, and you could be able to start full-time independent work.

It is possible to work for yourself and choose the customers and tasks you like best.

While variety can be your friend if you have the freedom to choose how that variety looks, overstimulation is still a threat to an HSP.

You might be able to use your skills in ways which make you feel good, keep you interested and happy, and decrease the risk of burnout by working with multiple customers or on different types of projects.

You can have the ideal HSP combination, doing meaningful work while having control over your workday. This is possible if you can do it in a space you own, on your schedule and with the people that you choose. This is true regardless your professional passion, expertise, or professional talent.

8. Pet groomer, trainer and caretaker

As pets are usually less demanding than people, it is common to only deal with one or two pets at once in these occupations.

For your own relaxation, it is a good idea to take a break from customers.

HSPs can calm animals down and win their trust. It is likely that spending time with animals will be less stressful than working with humans.

HSPs could benefit from their empathy and perceptiveness when caring for animals.

9. Hands-on work

This could be anything from building or producing handmade goods to designing interiors and cleaning out homes.

If you love working with your hands in a real environment and taking pride in creating beautiful things, or improving it, it may be a good fit for your personality. You may be able and willing to work at your own pace.

Just look for something that is HSP-friendly. You will likely be more successful if you make your own furniture than if the rest of the construction crew is busy.

For those with chemical sensitivities, eco-friendly cleaning may be a better option.

Particular details are important for sensitive people. If you find the right niche, it may be a useful option.

HSPs are quite valuable. HSPs are also more likely to face challenges at work than the average person. If they can find work that matches their abilities and caters to them, they could use their skills to make a difference and find fulfillment and enjoyment in their work.

If you are very sensitive, you might find a match with one of the nine professionals mentioned above. If your interests lie elsewhere you should be able find your ideal match using your unique insights and the suggested principles.

HSPs' Work Experience is Exhausting

Here are six ways HSPs can thrive at work in difficult and unpredictable situations.

1. A roadmap is essential.

HSPs pay attention to subtleties all around them. While this might seem overwhelming at first, it can be helpful to take some time after an event to record our thoughts and create a roadmap that can be broken down into smaller steps.

This makes it less overwhelming, easier to control, and ultimately, useful for managing oneself in difficult situations.

2. Get in touch.

HSPs are adept at building strong bonds with others. This type of connection may encourage team members to go beyond the call-of duty to accomplish their tasks.

You can make time to connect with colleagues and build trust during meetings. These meetings are increasingly being conducted via webcam. A theme or reflective question can help participants contribute more to the data and encourage a stronger sense for teamwork.

Your team will feel more competent and grounded in their work, even if it seems impossible at times.

3. Allocate time for dreaming.

HSPs can see beyond the normal and anticipate scenarios that are not possible. If these ideas are implemented effectively, they can lead to amazing achievements that are seen at the highest levels in a company.

Spend some time every week dreaming. Keep a record of your dreams, just as I suggested in my first piece. Later, dividing up specific tasks will ensure that bright, original ideas can be translated into tangible outcomes.

4. Your workspace should be kept clean and tidy.

You should make time for reorganization. HSPs are easily overwhelmed by clutter and other distractions that can drain your life force. Organization of your workspace throughout the day can provide you with much-needed, constant tranquility.

It doesn't matter if your office is not in your home. It is important to have a place in the room you can use only while you are working. Another option is to set up a portable, easy-to-clean table.

5. Give it purpose.

HSPs are motivated with "higher purposes" and want to prove that the things they care about matter. These higher goals are important for anyone who hasn't chosen a profession that is suited to their personality.

It will bring us back to our original motivations for picking the job if we take the time and consider how everyday actions can be linked to a higher purpose. Even though they don't always directly impact the bottom line of the company, it is important that we make sure to allocate time each day to tasks that are in support of our primary goal to contribute meaningfully.

6. Conserve energy.

Always remember to control your energy, not your time. This idea wasn't mine. Instead, you can watch this two-minute video from Gaining Traction. You have the ability to arrange your energy according you schedule.

HSPs need to fully grasp this concept. We are constantly processing so many things that we don't even know about, and we lose energy every minute.

Learn how to control your energies so you can focus on the activities and not the mess at the kitchen.

The six tactics above can help you to deal with difficult situations and be successful at work. Despite the world's tendency to favor loud personalities, our HSP superpowers enable us to operate instinctively, manage groups empathically and produce meaningful, actionable results.

It's not all about work. Do not neglect to schedule some downtime. You will do better at work if your are enthusiastic and ready to go.

Chapter 5: How to overcome impostor Syndrome and Perfectionism as an HSP

Many successful people have a secret that makes their achievements seem totally unworthy. They believe that luck was a key to their success.

Imposter syndrome describes a psychological condition in that you believe you're incompetent, inept or incapable of performing despite the evidence to the contrary.

It is a toxic flaming mass, for those who don't know. It can take many different forms depending upon the person's personality, upbringing, and current circumstances. It might help to identify the impostor in you to be able to effectively approach problems.

Expert on the topic Dr. Valerie Young arranged it into five subgroups, including the Expert, Perfectionist and Superwoman/Superman.

Dr. Young draws heavily on decades of research regarding the subject of high achievers emotions of imposter condition in her book, The Secret Thoughts of Successful Women - Why Capable People Suffer with the Imposter Condition and How to Thrive Despite.

Young discovered several "competence type" (internal guidelines that people with low confidence follow) through her research. It is not uncommon for this category of people to go unnoticed in a discussion. But, Young's analysis may be very valuable for identifying any patterns or negative tendencies that can prevent you from reaching all your potential.

By reading the following summary, you can check to see if any of Young's competencies are applicable to you. A few situations from your everyday life may also be relevant, and there are reflection questions.

1. The Obsessive

Perfectionism and imposter Syndrome often go hand in glove. Consider this: Perfectionists are often obsessed with perfection and feel inadequate when they don't achieve their goals.

This group, despite their ignorance, may also be control freaks. These people believe that they must perform the task themselves.

Do you think this applies to your situation? The following are some examples:

Did you ever get charged with micromanagement before?

Do you find delegating difficult? Do you get frustrated or disillusioned when delegating?

Are you tempted to dwell on your failures and guilt about "not being cut out" for your profession for many days?

Do you believe your work must be flawless all the time?

This personality is not satisfied with what they have achieved, because they believe they could have done even more. That is neither helpful nor productive. It is important to acknowledge and celebrate your achievements in order to avoid burnout and find fulfillment.

Accept mistakes and failures as part of the learning process. Do not force yourself into taking action before you have prepared. Do not force yourself to do the work you have been preparing for many weeks. Truth is, there won't be perfect timing or error-free labor. Accepting the change as soon as possible will make you more successful.

2. Superman or Superwoman

These people often find it difficult to maintain a competitive edge with their real-world peers. The problem is that this mask may only be temporary and can lead to job overload, which could have negative effects on their interpersonal relationships as well as their mental health.

Do you think this is the case for you?

Do you sometimes stay at work after the tasks are completed?

Do you feel stressed when you're not at work and find leisure useless?

Did you give up your passions and interests for your job?

Do you feel pressured to be more productive than your peers to establish your value, even though you may have many degrees or accomplishments?

False workaholics depend on the approval they get from work, not the work. You can learn to stop looking for approval from others. Even if you get the go-ahead from your employer, no one should be capable of making you feel better about your work than you. However, constructive criticism is something you can take seriously and still remain neutral.

As you learn to be more self-aware and have the ability to accept your limitations, you will be able taylor the pedal.

3. The Inborn Talent

Young states that this competency type assumes they must be "natural geniuses." Therefore, instead of looking at their efforts, these people judge their skills more on how easy and quick they are to do things. Also, people don't feel proud if it takes them awhile to do something.

Similar to perfectionists these imposters set very high internal standards. People who are naturally gifted evaluate themselves not only by their absurd standards, they also judge themselves on the quality of their completed tasks. If they aren't able to move quickly or fluidly, their alarm goes off.

Do you think this applies to your situation?

Are you used a doing well with little effort.

Are you someone who gets "straight A's" or "gold star" grades in all your activities?

Did someone tell you as a child that your intelligence was the best?

Are you able to handle things by yourself, or do you object the idea of having a mentor

Do you feel like you are losing confidence because of a setback that makes you feel shameful?

Do you find it difficult to take on a task you're not good at?

You can view yourself as a workman in progress if this is something you would like to discuss. Everyone, even the most self-assured, needs to continue learning new skills and developing existing ones in order achieve greatness. Instead of feeling guilty if you fail to live up to your expectations, focus on the positive habits that you can cultivate over time.

You can improve your ability to present if you want to have an impact at work.

4. The Soloist

Soloists are those who fear being exposed as phonies by Young. Independent living is fine, but you shouldn't be so independent that you don't accept help in order to prove your value.

Do you think this is the case for you? The following are some examples:

Do you believe that you are obligated to complete tasks on your own?

I don't need to be helped by anyone. You sound like that?

What are your needs as a project manager?

Recognize it is acceptable to ask for assistance when needed. Ask your coworker for help if you don't know how to do something. If you are having trouble coming up a solution, ask your boss or a career coach.

5. The Expert

Experts rate their competence on the basis of "what" as well as "how many" they are capable or know. Because they don't think they are competent enough, they worry about their lack of expertise or experience.

Are you willing to apply for jobs even though you don't meet the education requirements?

Do you look for training opportunities and certificates to help you succeed?

Can you relate to feeling like you don't know "enough" even though you've been in the same position for a while.

Do you cringe when someone calls your an expert?

You always have more to learn. Expanding your skills will help you to grow professionally and be more competitive in the job marketplace. The propensity to not stop learning can lead to procrastination if it's taken to the extreme.

Get started on your just-in time learning skills. This is learning a skill as you need it.

You can discover your inner genius by mentoring or volunteering with younger colleagues. Share your knowledge to benefit others as well as your own self-healing from emotions associated with fraud.

You are not the only one feeling insecure, no matter what your job title. Research suggests that at least 70% of employees suffer from impostor's syndrome at some point in their careers.

If you feel this way about your job or your life, chances are you have at least once attributed it to luck, charm, connections or another uncontrollable force.

This is unjust and cruel! You can use today to acknowledge and appreciate your strengths.

Chapter 6: How to Thrive when you're a Highly Sensitive parent.

Being sensitive may make parenting more difficult. Parents who are hypersensitive to children are often overwhelmed by their need for stimulation, noise, cleanliness, dependency, and constant stimulation.

Since becoming a mother, I've struggled with this. (It's not surprising that one of my daughters finds it hilarious to scream, simply because it makes mother nuts.)

My sensitive nature makes it hard for me to be calm, present, and patient with my kids when things are chaotic. I feel the need to retreat into the silent bathroom and hide from the chaos, disruption, and turmoil that surrounds me when my children are around.

Being sensitive isn't all bad. Let's talk about some of the advantages and disadvantages that an HSP could face.

Benefits of being sensitive parents

You may find parenting more rewarding if your children are sensitive.

High-sensitivity parents are highly organized. Parents with high sensitivity levels are meticulous and organized. They also have the propensity for being efficient and effective. While we don't always achieve perfection, it is possible to feel overwhelmed and not be able to complete tasks effectively.

Children who have sensitive parents tend to be more aware of their needs than the average parent. It helps them feel secure and loved. High-sensitivity parents are often able predict their children's needs before they ever speak. Being able to recognize the tiny signals that our children send us can help us react quickly and effectively. This allows us to foster trust, kinship and healthy attachment between child and parent.

Dr. Aron asserts that HSPs are naturals with newborns, as we often get along nicely with young children and animals who are unable or unwilling to communicate verbally. They are comfortable and happy because they believe we are in sync. When they speak, we often pause and think before responding, so that we can model such behaviour for our children.

Parents with high levels sensitivity should be aware of what makes each child unique and special. Dr. Aron believes that HSPs are more apt to recognize the individual characteristics of their children and treat them as such. Children feel more confident, respected, and worthy as a result.

High parental sensitivity. Parents who are HS parents have experienced everything, the great, the bad, and everything in between. Our children's success is a source of great satisfaction for us, and we enjoy spending time with our families. Parenthood brings us all the joys, happiness, and love that comes with it. Dr. Aron says that parents with high levels of sensitive children often think parenting is "possibly better rewarding," which can keep them working through the thick and thin.

Being sensitive to your child's needs is a difficult job. It's all hard.

Kidding... (sort of).

There is almost no downtime.

A parent works nonstop. No matter what you do, you are still a parent. This means that you should be always active. This means that you must be available even when sleeping. There are good chances that even though we aren't near our children, we are still thinking about them. The mental strain is real and exhausting.

Children are naturally lively. They are very energetic and love being surrounded by attention. It can be hard for anyone to understand, but it is more difficult for parents who are sensitive. According to Dr. Aron, our children might "burn us all out, making us irritated and even out-ofcontrol furious in short-term as well as sad about a potential future of chronic hyperarousal."

These children may be more sensitive if they are "deeply feeling," as Dr. Becky Kenndey describes them. These children can be wildly dysregulated, and they often drive their parents crazy.

Dr. Becky explains that DFK parents need clarity and confidence in their approach because of the delay between intervention and its effect. So you will have to deal with lots of "Is this my youngster taking in?" questions. You will also have to ask the question, "Is this making any difference?" Keep in mind that the difficulty you face when raising a DFK is not due to your failing, but because the situation is difficult.

Additionally, she believes it is difficult for parents to help their children who are profoundly emotional navigate their feelings. Parents often struggle with managing their own strong emotions as can be the case with HSPs. Good Inside has excellent advice on how to raise DFKs. Her advice is not only for HSPs, but also for those who are emotionally fragile.

It is common for parents to be sensitive. Yes, it was advantageous. However, it is possible to feel all of the negative emotions while fully experiencing the positive. Parents who are extremely sensitive experience all emotions of their children, including conflict and happiness. Any of the emotional, mental, and physical pains our children experience can make us feel physically sick, even though it may help us become better empathizers.

One example is when one of my kids suffers from separation anxiety at drop-off school. I feel deeply guilty for having coaxed them to their classroom. I can't stop crying and it can become quite crippling. To get the tension out it takes me time and an email to the teacher.

Losing your cool. This happens quite often and is almost always followed by a deep sense of guilt. I weep for the children and apologize, but the cycle keeps going. Dr. Aron stated that parents who have children in high school need to monitor their emotional state. This is particularly true when their children are feeling fatigued or overwhelmed. This is very similar to what happens with extremely emotional children (as I mentioned earlier).

DFK can't control their strong emotions. They get overwhelmed, embarrassed, and overwhelmed by them. It makes perfect sense that many of the highly sensitive parents were themselves very emotional children and weren't given the right support or the skills needed to manage those strong emotions.

Parental regret. It's not just guilt we've been talking about, but very sensitive parents can experience it. When parents are sensitive, they often feel shame and guilt when they make mistakes in parenting, lose their tempers, have to take a break from mental health, neglect their children, or don't prioritize their own needs. I cannot tell you how many times I lay down in bed at the end, mentally adding up all my parenting mistakes and taking self-care breaks, feeling like a failure.

Manage Life as a Highly Sensitive Parents:

Yes, it is difficult to be sensitive with a child. But, it is not impossible. With the right strategies and tips, you can increase your ability to be present for your children as well as yourself. You can be sensitive and manage your parenting by using the following tips.

Time to yourself. I've spoken before about how terrible I used to feel about parenting and needing help. However, I learned the hard way that taking breaks is good for my health and energy. I am a happier, calmer, more patient, present, and more present parent.

Dr. Aron agrees. Dr. Aron agrees. Similar to other difficulties, it is impossible to compare yourself with others who are HSPs. It is important to emphasize this point. If you do not love being a parent and are afraid of having to deal with another day with your child, seek help.

This topic deserves my attention. I felt insecure and guilty that I needed help. It took me many years, counseling, and learning about what it meant to be a HSP to see that my needs were different than those of other parents. If this is you let all of the shame, humiliation, guilt, and sorrow associated feeling insufficient go. It's not worthwhile and it's not fair for you or your children.

You are the parent that your children need. Keep this in mind. You'll be more successful in this job by taking breaks and asking for assistance.

Establish limits: Know your boundaries. A different plan is available if you know that you can't take all your children to the grocery shopping because they are disruptive and throw things in the cart without you looking. Instacart (or other delivery services) may deliver your groceries to you. A friend, spouse or parent can help. Watch your kids as you shop. Or, bring them along.

Whatever you do, don't compare yourself to others. Release any guilt or shame that you may feel in this regard.

The Seleni Institute, an organization that supports the emotional health and well-being of families, advises that setting clear boundaries is key to maintaining your emotional and physical well-being. Although it is tempting to push yourself beyond your limits, it can cause headaches and even chronic weariness. You should listen to your body when you need to rethink.

Recognize and love who you really are. Your brain wired in such an efficient way that it makes your sensitive. As an inherent characteristic, you were born with it. You feel everything deeply and continuously. This is not a reflection of you. You may have heard it said that others should "toughen you up" or "develop thicker pores" during your entire life.

But you'll be able to see that being a high-skilled person (HSP) is not just a gift.

Self-Care. Take the necessary steps for you to take care of your own health. Do not drown - you will not be able to properly or at all care for your children. It is important to always wear your oxygen mask before helping others.

Attain similar goals: It is possible to search Google or Facebook for HSP support groups and resources. It's easy to feel isolated when you meet people who share your very sensitive qualities and can relate. We are certain that there are many more HSPs around than you think.

If needed, get expert assistance. Therapy benefits everyone. Dr. Elaine Aron keeps an up-to-date list of occupations in each state that deal with mental health. Sensitivity HSP-aware

HSP-focused counselors can even provide virtual treatment in the privacy of their clients' homes. Sensory processing therapy and occupational therapy are other useful options.

Five Strategies for Overwhelm

Five full breathes: You shouldn't underestimate the importance of taking a few deep belly inhalations to relieve tension. When I feel stressed, my favorite breathing method is the 4-7-8 technique. This involves taking a big inhale and counting up to 4, while holding it for 7 counts. Next, take a slow exhale while counting down to 8. I feel relieved.

Be active: Any form of exercise, from a five-minute yoga break to a block stroll, increases the production and release of happy endorphins. This reduces stress, overload, anxiety, and panic. My kids find it hilarious (and odd) that I perform jumping jacks right in the middle my kitchen.

You should get rid of the batteries in the toys for your children. Even better, don't give your children items that are loud, bright or stimulating. They won't be needed by you either.

Engage with nature frequently: Research has shown that spending time in the natural world (or even just listening for sounds that resemble it) is a great way to connect with nature. It can improve your mood, well-being and mental health.

The cruise ship director job is over. You don't have the obligation to entertain your children constantly. They can play on their own for a while; this is even a good thing. Relax and let go of any guilt. Enjoy a cup o' tea in the other area, enjoy your favorite podcast, or just dance to your favorite music. Your kids don't need you to be around them 24/7. In fact, I have been known to go to the closet or bathroom for a short time to get a "breathing room").

If you take care of yourself, your children will learn how important it is to have boundaries and practice self-care.

Reading this essay can help you gain a better understanding of the unique traits and personality you have, especially if you consider yourself to be sensitive.

High sensitivity can lead a person to feel exhausted or overstimulated. For example, you might be overwhelmed by your children singing, dancing, light-up toys and other lights. You may also experience constant bickering, random, ear-piercing noises, and many other emotional and physical needs.

You are extraordinarily sensitive about your children's needs, wants, sufferings, joys and excitements.

This is what your children will always remember. That's something my children value about me. What about the rest of it? You become more fascinating, complex and deeply aware. As a result you are a better parent and person. That's pretty incredible.

Chapter 7: Social Media Detoxes for an HSP are Beneficial

In today's digital world, being on social media has become a standard. If you don't use Facebook, Twitter, or Instagram, you are living under a rock. Social media has a significant impact on our lives today, but it's also possible to do just about anything via it. From connecting with friends to learning to cook to online shopping, to ordering groceries.

This doesn't mean you shouldn't use your phone as much as you like. It is important to avoid social media.

What exactly is a "social media cleaning"? It is a process that involves completely avoiding all social media sites, and also putting your phone down. A social media detox can be done for a day or week by psychologists. It is believed to boost happiness and mental function.

And this is what I advise you to do. You know by now that using social media is not good for your mental well-being. While social media is great for interacting with others and staying in touch, it can also cause people to have a different view of reality. After all, you're only viewing the highlights in other peoples' lives. While it may be hard to believe that you are addicted social media, think about how often your phone is checked each day. This is depressing.

However, you should not allow such a habit to continue. It is quite simple to just delete all the applications that keep us busy every day.

Why would you do that? These five wonderful things will be possible because of your digital fast.

You'll feel more confident. Your confidence will rise if you regularly see someone with a "perfect figure", "beautiful face", or "successful life". You begin to compare yourself to them and believe you are always lacking. We are here to affirm that social media doesn't reflect reality. It is important to start appreciating yourself for what you are, rather than trying to copy someone you have seen online.

A digital detox can help you to let go of comparisons and allow you to spend more time doing things that bring you joy.

Unique moments will be worth your attention. Humans are inclined to give the past less attention than it deserves, and to be more focused on the future. Individuals want more. It is possible that we spend too much of our time worrying about the lives of others, rather than enjoying our own unique moments.

If you are ever faced with something new, resist the urge not to share it on social networks and instead just enjoy the moment.

You'll be less anxious. You will feel less anxious. This can cause excessive checking, worrying, and posting.

By taking a vacation, you may be able to stop the vicious cycle.

You'll get back in touch. Despite the absurdity of it, you'll be more social. Relationships can only develop and last if they are built on face-to–face communication. Although social media might seem to be a great tool for friendship and connection, quality time is still the key to any successful relationship.

Additionally, you'll have more free time. How often have we all wished we had more time for ourselves? Therefore, you shouldn't include time spent on your phone as it doesn't serve any purpose for you.

One person could spend up to two hours daily on social media. This time could be better used for other productive and more worthwhile endeavors. Use those two hours for something creative. You'll feel 10x more satisfied and fuller!

Nearly everyone is dependent upon social media. You don't have to change your routine. Even though you may be scared to try taking a break, you must do it for your own good. Your happiness is your responsibility.

Do you find social media a time sapper or a worry-inducing tool? I'll be discussing more than 100 options for replacing social media.

According to various surveys, most people scroll through social networks for hours each day.

This is what many people end up doing for their day.

You check Facebook or Instagram first thing in the morning when you get up from your bed.

You could then contemplate it while eating breakfast.

When you arrive at your job, you make sure to check it again.

During lunch you check out Facebook or Instagram.

In between lectures, peruse your feed (or even in class).

After work, you can start over.

Before going to bed.

I am aware that there are certain people who will get up in the middle night to check social networks.

Seriously, you likely spend all day on social networking and your phone.

I want to talk about many different activities that you can engage in, rather than using social networking.

These principles are still applicable if you want to watch less TV.

If you feel that you don't reach your goals or are being constantly pressured to make time, analyze how much time is wasted each day.

Your time spent on Facebook, Instagram, Twitter and all your other social media accounts might not be obvious to you.

When you realize how much time social media is wasting, I encourage you to get some back.

More than 100 activities can be used to replace your social networking.

Never get out the bedside table or rise from your phone.

I am trying my best to improve. I don't carry my laptop to bed anymore, but I need it to be put down. It is very difficult not to use social media.

After a set time, I've come to know people who don't check their phones again until the morning. I will think about this until the morning. This should be done by more people, including me.

It is possible to regain control and manage your life by simply changing one thing.

Learn new things, expand your horizons.

While it might be difficult at first to not use social media, you will soon find that you are able to try new activities and enjoy unique experiences. You can try things you never imagined and do things you always wanted to.

There is always something new to see and discover. You could engage in a multitude of activities that will enrich your life, make you better and help you to grow. If you don't try some, you won't discover what your talents are. You may discover a new talent, or even an interest.

Try these activities instead of just scrolling through the social media.

Do you get tired of repeating the same recipes? Learning how to cook a dish out of your comfort zones is one of the best things you can do without social media.

Listen to music or create a music list.

Consider listening to a podcast. There are many podcasts that can be used to teach, entertain, or instruct. You may choose.

Write down your ideas in a journal.

Setting goals can help you grow. These objectives can be helpful in your growth.

Travel with friends and family. While it might be time-consuming, you can enjoy exploring new places while researching. A staycation can be the most affordable option.

Color and have fun. There are coloring books for adults!

Visit a gallery. What is the most recent time you have visited a museum?

You can check out the library. You can loan books or movies to borrow, which you can then get back and enjoy with your family or friends at home. In some libraries, you can also borrow state and national park permits, camping gear, or other items.

Join a reading group

Learn new knowledge. Learn how to do many different activities, including knitting, crocheting and dancing.

Read a blog, or read a book. If you're looking for something to do, reading may be a better choice than social media.

Become bilingual. You can attend classes, read books, and utilize applications.

Attend a concert. You can even find free concerts in the area.

Find out how to invest. Your money wouldn't be earning anything if you weren't investing.

Find alternatives to social media and spend more outdoor time.

Being outside and physically active are the best things to do rather than using social media.

This could improve your mental, physical, and general well-being.

Below is a quick list of outdoor activities you could do instead of using social media.

Go for a bike ride.

Take a hike.

Try yoga.

Meditate.

Geocache.

Try canoeing, kayaking, or both.

Rock climbing is a great option.

Take a walk, even if it's only around your neighborhood.

Have fun with you pet.

Go swimming.

Observe the night skies.

Catch fish.

You can explore new areas in your city.

Make sure to camp.

Enjoy a barbecue

A bonfire is a great idea.

You can walk around the city.

Be aware of the sunrise and the sunset.

Gather your friends and go outside for a scavenger search.

You can find free places to see in your locality.

You can become a marathon-ready.

Increase your output.

You might be able to make time for other things in your life if you either stop using it altogether or reduce how long you spend on it.

Many of these can increase productivity, which will allow you to work faster overall.

By removing yourself from social media, you can save time. You may also be able to use that time to make more time.

Instead of using social networks, you can try these activities that will increase productivity.

Even if the space is just a drawer, organize it.

This is one option to make your money and expenses more manageable than social media.

Initiate a task to your to-do lists.

You can use a bullet notebook to organize your week and days in a fun and engaging way.

You should look for ways to improve your processes.

Get ready to take on the mountain.

Weekly food program.

Make sure to wash your dishes.

Get into your bed

Eliminate the waste.

Automate your invoice payments with autopay

You can save money by finding ways to reduce costs.

There are many other activities you can do instead of using social networks. You'll feel amazing if you take the time to do things that you don't often have the time for.

Do some housework, while you're away from social media.

Almost every home has a list with tasks to complete.

However, using social media to delay tasks may help. Now it's time that you've stopped this, it's now time to get on with the task at hand.

Here are some other activities you could do at home, instead of using social networks:

Organize. You could organize your files, drawers or crafts, your basement, and/or attic.

.

Declutter: You can get rid of most clutter.

Sort through your pantry.

DIY initiatives: Everybody has a project in mind. It's time to get started.

Painting your home is a must.

Select a room to clean.

Report your plants and prune them.

Enjoy great food by taking your time. It's hard to imagine a better way of eating.

Move your furniture around. This could make your home feel more spacious and clean.

Routine upkeep for your house. It's almost impossible to find something that doesn't involve upkeep for your home.

You should consider doing some home improvement. A majority of homeowners have damaged things in their homes. Spend some time fixing it!

Your financial position should be improved. Financial freedom is when you're able to enjoy your life and not have to worry about money. It happens when you are able to pursue your passion without worrying too much about money.

A well-maintained emergency fund can help you avoid worrying about an unexpected bill. It is not necessary to be financially independent. It is about your level and spending habits, financial goals, and how much you are able to save.

It is much better to use social media than to try to boost your wealth!

launch a garden. Fresh food is the best kind of cuisine.

Help people and the surrounding environment find social media substitutions.

There are so much you can do to improve the world.

Random acts or kindness can have a positive impact on everyone. Random acts and acts of kindness can help others, but they are also good for you.

It doesn't really matter how small the gesture, it will make a significant difference.

Even the smallest of things can transform someone's mood and make their day better!

This list of activities you can do instead of using social networks will make you, and your family, happy.

Donate household goods. A second option is to donate something for every new item that you bring home. Contribute a shirt to every shirt you buy.

Volunteer in a field that interests you.

All people you come in contact with should say hello and smile. I am always grateful when people share their kindness with me.

Don't be afraid to give your blood.

Take along a trash bag and stuff it with all the rubbish you see on your walks.

You can take care of your pet. You might consider adopting a new pet if you're able.

Consider donating to a new charity.

Read books in a library or hospital.

Join the Big Brother/Big Sister program.

Prepare ready-to–go bags for those who are less fortunate. If you are able to help the homeless, put small packets or dog food in a bag.

Consider strategies that will increase your income.

I am a big believer in generating additional income. It can change your life.

Your financial health will improve, both now and into the future.

You will be amazed at how much free time you have when you stop using social media. You may have as many as 10-20 hours per week available to you to work on increasing your income.

These are some other ways to make extra money than using social media.

Respond to polls. I endorse Swagbucks. Survey Junkie. Pinecone Research. Branded Surveys. Participating in these surveys and using them are free. Reviewing products and participating in surveys can earn you compensation. You can earn more money by signing up for as many surveys and products as you like.

You could consider dog walking, pet sitting, or pet-sitting to earn extra cash. Rover is an excellent way to begin your career as a dog walker or pet caregiver.

You should start a website: This is my number one recommendation for making money. It is possible to proofread and edit text. Editors are needed for websites. It doesn't really matter how many times someone has read the same piece of material, it always seems to go missing. If you're a grammar nerd, this can be a great way for you to make money.

Photographing: Are you passionate about taking pictures? It is possible to make money by working as a wedding, portrait, event or other type of photographer. Learn more about how to start a food blog and earn over $50,000 per annum, as well How to make $25,000 to $45,000 per year as a new photographer.

Garage sale: This is a fantastic way to spend your free time and get rid off all the junk that has been gathering around your home.

Facebook advertising manager for local businesses: Did you realize that you might earn between $1,000 and $2,000 more per month by managing Facebook ads? This is the complete interview. How to Use Facebook to Earn $1,000 More in Your Time.

Bookkeeper Business Academy founder Ben shows you how you might be able to take up bookkeeping. Ben's online accounting training helps individuals to start or grow their bookkeeping companies. And guess what? You don't need to have any prior experience. This could be a fantastic way to find work, instead of browsing social media. Learn more on How to Make Money From Home While Working as a Bookkeeper.

Amazon selling: Set up an Amazon FBA company to make your time productive. Jane Huston of The Selling Family shows you how to sell on Amazon. I consider her a friend, and she has achieved amazing feats. Jane's family was able to earn over six figures the first year they owned their Amazon FBA company. Jane worked a total of less than 20 hour per week.

This is one option if you don't want to use social media for your search for a new job or side gig.

Deliver meals or deliver goods: A growing number of people use food delivery services. There are many businesses in which you might work, including DoorDash

(UberEats), Shipt (Shipt), and UberEats (Shipt).

Blood, plasma, eggs, etc. They can be donated or sold. These items can all be sold or donated for a profit. You will definitely increase your income.

Mysterious shopping: Mystery shopping is an alternative to social media. Your restaurant or retail purchase can result in you being compensated. A few years back I did a lot in mystery shopping to make more money. I was paid between $150 to $200 per month for mystery-shopping, plus free meals, cosmetics and other things.

Bestmark was the only company that I used for mystery shopping. However, there are many other mystery shopping businesses that you can trust.

Look through your closet and home for gently used items, then make an offer to sell them online. Poshmark, Facebook

Marketplace, or other platforms could earn you extra cash.

You don't have only to use social networks to increase your income. There are many different activities that you could engage in.

You can improve your relationships with those around you.

You can potentially use the time you save using less social media to increase your connections with people you care about.

Many people are content to use their phones only when they're out with friends and families, taking part in activities, or doing nothing else. This could cause you to lose touch with the people that matter most to your heart.

But, with more time, your bonds may strengthen with close friends, family, and even complete strangers.

It is possible to reclaim your life, and increase your relationships, by learning how to make more use of social media. You never know when someone might be interested in reaching out to you.

These are some activities that can help you build relationships with your friends and family through social media.

Contact a family member. It could be you, or someone else, that needs to be reached right away. Although everyone text these days, I prefer to make phone calls. It's weird to receive so few phone calls after so many years.

Send a thank-you note or handwritten letter to someone.

Spending time doing this may prove to be beneficial.

Organise a movie night. It is fun and inexpensive to spend time with loved ones.

Visit a family member or friend in person. Quality time is something that can't be rushed. You can schedule a video conference call with them if they are far away.

You can volunteer together with a friend. If you are both interested in the same project, it can help you to strengthen your friendship.

Get together. It may be a good idea to gather everyone together and catch up.

.

You can start an accountability team with a friend. You can meet with a buddy once per week to check in and discuss your progress towards your goals.

Take the time to cook dinner for someone special. You can make a difference whether you're a friend who just welcomed a child or you know someone who struggles.

Speak to someone from the outside. When we are out in public, we often look at our phones instead of paying attention to what is happening around us. You might start a conversation. You never know who you will meet, or how eager someone might be to speak with you.

What can you do with a phone without social media but not Facebook?

It's quite funny that this is such a common query. Your phone can do much more than simply use social media.

You can make use of your calendar, learn a new language, or make phone calls (one the first things you can do on a smartphone instead of using social media), as well as many other activities.

Can social media make me happier

While I do not advocate that you abandon all social media, it is possible to make a living from it. Even though it is possible that you will be happier spending less time on social networking sites.

How do I pass the time if I don't use social media?

There are many things you can do offline to keep yourself entertained, as you'll see in the list.

Social media is essential in today's modern world. You can choose a few. You are most likely living under a rock, if you don't use Facebook, Twitter, or Instagram.

Social media has a significant impact on our lives today, but it is also possible to do just about anything via it. From connecting with friends to learning to cook to shopping online, to making connections and sharing your thoughts.

This doesn't mean you shouldn't use your phone as much as you like. It is important to avoid social media.

Find alternatives to social media and spend more outdoor time.

Enjoy the items on this list!

Chapter 8: Living with high sensitivity

It is possible that this book has made you feel too sensitive or thought you were crazy. You may have been told not to listen to too much environmental noise. You might even be told by the environment that being sensitive is a negative trait. Some people feel that they have to overcome or correct a character "defect" to be accepted. High-sensitivity people are more creative, sensitive and compassionate than the rest of society. All of these qualities deserve to be celebrated.

High-sensitivity people may become easily overwhelmed, resistant to change, and often feel uneasy. These emotions can be challenging to manage and can cause a lot of problems in one's daily life. You can deal with these issues by accepting your individuality and looking for ways to maximize your talents while working around your limitations.

What is High Sensitivity?

The person who is highly sensitive is one who has a deep understanding of and an acute response to both external and inner stimuli. It's a personality trait called sensory processing sensitivity. The central nervous system is highly sensitive to mental, social, and physical stimuli.

HSPs are more emotionally and physically sensitive than others. The normal personality characteristic of high sensitivity is one that is healthy and accepted. However, as with all personality characteristics, there are benefits and disadvantages.

HSPs react more emotionally to life experiences than the average individual. They are more sensitive towards external information which makes it more difficult for HSPs to cope with noisy noises and large crowds. Popular author Elaine Aron has attributed high sensitivity to 15-20% of the population.

HSPs are born with a genetic difference that gives them a greater understanding of subtleties and information processing. HSPs are more creative, intuitive and resourceful than other people. However, they can be more susceptible to feeling stressed out and overwhelmed. The most sensitive person will likely be overwhelmed with empathy, emotion and accurate reading of social situations. HSPs are extremely aware of their surroundings.

Highly sensitive people are more relaxed and enjoy taking in the subtleties of life at a slower pace. HSPs may find it more enjoyable to smell their morning coffee and see the world from their window, rather than enjoying loud music or crowds. This makes sense to those who are sensitive to overstimulation. Small pleasures and a lighter routine allow them the freedom to achieve their best without feeling overwhelmed.

It is important to know that although sensitivity has been widely recognized as a personality trait, the American Psychological Association still doesn't officially recognize it as one its Big Five personality traits.

Common Signs That a Person Is Highly Sensitive is

Each HSP experience is different depending on their life stage. These are the most obvious and prominent symptoms that an extremely sensitive person may experience. Check out these symptoms and see if they are familiar to you.

You are scared of change.

HSPs find it easy to settle into their routines, as they are less stimulated than new ones. HSPs are susceptible to being destroyed by change. HSPs could experience more stress if they have to meet new people or receive a promotion. HSPs often take longer to adjust to new situations than other types of people.

You may have been misunderstood.

It is common to misunderstand the term "high sensitive" when you are speaking of someone who has high sensitivity. Perhaps you were called "shy" or anxious, even though it was not true.

You're unable to handle criticism

HSPs consider words to be extremely important. While positive words can take them off the ground, harsh words can send their confidence plummeting. Criticism can strike as hard as a dagger. Negative consequences can prove toxic for someone who is sensitive.

Time constraints cause you stress.

Timed school tests made you anxious and could even make it impossible to perform normally. Adults often feel overwhelmed by too many tasks and limited time. Time pressure is not a friend.

You often feel anxious.

When someone walks up to you, you will jump like a scared kitten. Many HSPs have strong "startle reflex," which happens when their nervous systems activate even in nonthreatening circumstances.

You tend to withdraw the most.

No matter if you're an extrovert/introvert, you still need some downtime. You will often retreat to a darkened and quiet space after a long day. This allows you to lower your stimulation level, relax your senses, and recharge.

All forms of cruelty and violence are detested.

While everyone hates cruelty and violence, those with high levels of sensitive skin may find it particularly distressing. An HSP is someone who finds it difficult to watch scary or violent movies without feeling sick or dizzy. HSPs will not tolerate any news about animal cruelty, or other horrendous acts.

Emotional overload can make you exhausted.

Highly sensitive people tend to "soak in" other people's emotions. HSPs often can feel the mood in a room when they walk into it. Because people with high levels of sensitivities are sensitive to subtleties such voice tone, facial expressions, and linguistics that others might overlook, this is not uncommon. HSPs can be tolerant of others' feelings, thanks to their natural capacity for empathy. High levels of sensitivity can lead to emotional stress in people who are sensitive.

You have a conflict problem.

You are very aware of any conflict or friction in your close relationships. Many HSPs experience bodily discomfort during argument times. High-sensitive people are more sensitive than others and avoid conflict. They will say or do anything to please the other person if it causes internal distress.

You become flustered when you hear loud noises.

A motorcycle, helicopter, or fire engine roaring through the window can shake up an HSP.

You have a lower tolerance of physical pain.

Many types and degrees of pain, such a headache, bodily aches, or wounds, are more painful for HSPs that they are for non-HSPs.

HSPs can experience positive traits, despite the negative symptoms. These are some of the most common:

Beauty is deeply moving.

Beautiful music, delicious food, rich scents, exquisite artwork and beautiful meals all have a profound influence on you. The way the wind picks up the leaves during the fall sun can transport you to a state that is almost trance-like, or it may cause you to be completely absorbed by certain sounds and music. It's difficult to imagine why beauty doesn't move others as much as you do.

Your clothes are very important.

Always be conscious of what clothing you are wearing. Wearing restrictive clothing could cause irritation. It is possible for non-HSPs to dislike the same thing. However, an HSP carefully selects their clothing so that they do not get it.

Your curiosity is excessive.

HSPs constantly search for answers to the most pressing issues in life. These individuals are often confused about how things turned out and what their function in this entire situation is. It is possible that you have wondered why other people don't find the same fascination with the mysteries of human nature or the world.

You should think deeply.

HSP is founded on deep internal processing. This means you can think more about your experience. This also means you are more likely to think in negative ways. You might find yourself replaying too many events in your mind or spiraling into unsettling thoughts.

Chapter 9: The Impact of Childhood Neglect

If you consider your self highly sensitive, then you should understand that your childhood experiences have a huge impact on how you feel as an adult. Although you may be more affected than others by your difficult childhood, this doesn't mean you shouldn't or should not try to mitigate those effects.

Although high sensitivity is considered a "nature" rather than "nurture" trait it can still have an effect on your overall well being. Your interactions with the environment will determine how sensitive you are. Sensitivity doesn't "improve" or decrease. As an example, if you were highly sensitive as a child and your intelligence was valued and rewarded, then you are more likely be that way as an adult.

But if your sensitive childhood experiences made you embarrassed, it is possible that you don't know how to manage your sensitive adult self. You may find yourself becoming more critical of your own flaws if you keep your eyes on them.

What happens when the trait of being valued is not valued or stressed?

Studies have shown that emotional neglect is a common outcome of families with relatively stable incomes. This happens because they fail to recognize and respond to their children's needs. This can be very harmful for any child. However, sensitive children are more at risk. One feels empty and unappreciated when one's emotions aren't met.

One of the most common causes of child neglect is when a parent fails to meet their child's emotional and physical needs. While this neglect may not seem serious at first glance, it can lead to severe loneliness and emotional or physical abuse. Because of this, HSPs can grow up with deep-rooted feelings of shame and regret.

These findings are due in part to the fact that HSPs use emotions first language. The family that does not understand their child's emotions is not speaking the language. They are not able to express their feelings, but they will try to suppress or hide the emotions of others. Simply put, they are trying to shut down their HSP child's true self. Children who have been subject to emotional neglect will learn that asking someone for help can lead them to being rejected or labeled weak. Children with high-strung personalities (HSP) must learn to advocate on their own behalf in a world that does not often understand them.

It shouldn't surprise that children with low self-esteem tend to be distrustful and devalue their own abilities. Parents who are not able to validate or recognize their child's strengths may see their child's shyness a problem and force their child to feel secure.

HSPs generally have trouble with criticism. This is often stressful for children. Children with high functioning autism (HFA), do not get effective feedback if their parents have suffered emotional neglect. If children have never seen these strategies in practice at home, it's unrealistic to expect them to learn the appropriate coping techniques.

A child who is extremely sensitive will need to be accommodated by their parents if they show compassion. If they don't, the parents may feel that the child is exaggerating. They might become frustrated with them. Overcomed children may experience anxiety and increased stress.

Emotional neglect in childhood doesn't disappear as you get older. As adults carry it into adulthood, it can impact everything HSPs touch, such as relationships, self-image, mental well being, and even their relationships. HSPs recovering from neglect often keep their emotions in check, or may become "numb", due to their emotional walled nature. Highly sensitive people only can express their emotions (or withdraw) when they are overwhelmed.

It's possible to correct emotional neglect from childhood. As an adult HSP you should be capable of expressing your emotions in everyday conversations. As you start treating yourself with respect & dignity, people around you will begin to respond in a different manner to you. Once they get the chance to get to know each other, they can begin to understand your personality and feelings.

More importantly, they start to focus on you.

Chapter 10: Quiz to Assess Yourself

You may still not be sure if you are HSP after reviewing the symptoms and characteristics. Below is a quick quiz that will help determine your status.

Answer each statement according to how you feel. Answer "yes" to a statement that is somewhat true. If it isn't true, or it isn't true at all, answer "no".

Extremely hungry can trigger a strong reaction within me which hinders my ability concentrate and maintain positive attitudes.

Yes ____.

When I experience change in my personal and professional lives, my nerves can get jittery.

Yes ____.

Disconcerting stimuli such flashing lights and strong odors or sirens are easy to overwhelm me.

Yes ___.

I consider my self to be a person with high moral character.

Yes ___.

I find it easy to be surprised at any time.

Yes ___.

I find it irritating when I have to do too much at the same.

Yes ___.

Beautiful artwork, beautiful smells, sounds and delicious tastes are what pique my curiosity and make me appreciate them more.

Yes ___.

I am a planner and try to avoid stressful or overwhelming situations.

Yes ___.

Extreme stimuli, like loud noises or chaotic scenes, make it uncomfortable.

Yes ___.

My moods and thoughts can be affected by those around me.

Yes ___.

I am extremely sensitive to pain and discomfort.

Yes ___.

When stressed, I need to go back to my bed.

Yes ___.

If you answered 'yes to six or greater of these statements, then your most likely highly sensitive.

Due to your sensitive nature, you may sometimes feel misunderstood. All HSPs have to deal with overstimulation or overwhelm from time to time. HSPs are more sensitive to their environment, no matter how supportive or negative. This can make it seem like being extremely sensitive can be both a blessing (or a curse) at times in your life. But, you should know that testing as a sensitive person is not just natural and healthy, but is also a powerful skill set.

Because of their strong emotions, such as anxiety, joy or joy, highly sensitive people tend not to take the time to consider everything. This intense thinking can lead to overwhelming feelings, especially if you're experiencing negative emotions. You need to be able to regulate your emotions.

What is emotional regulation and what does it do?

Emotional regulation is a process that we all use intuitively or unconsciously in our daily lives to control our mood. A stroll in the park might be a good idea if you feel angry. You may not want to make a fool of yourself if you find something funny. These kinds of responses are examples emotional regulation.

Be aware that the fundamental definition of emotional regulation says that this behavior is unconscious. Our actions are most likely learned as children or adopted from stressful situations. It is not common for everyone to learn how to deal with adversity and regulate their emotions from a young age. Many HSPs have difficulty developing an understanding of emotion regulation as adults due to a lack of self-regulation skills from childhood.

Because they are able to see the environment more clearly, negative emotions can be more difficult for people with high sensitivity. An HSP's brain is more active than that of non-HSPs and can cause erratic emotion fluctuations. HSPs can feel like they're on a rollercoaster when dealing with major life changes. The prospect of dealing with life changes can make you feel happy one minute and then anxious the next.

While positive emotions can be a joy, it can become overwhelming when you have to deal with negative emotions. An example of this is when you become overwhelmed by anxiety.

Many highly sensitive people feel they have a problem because of these extreme feelings. HSPs can deal with "more emotions" because they take in other peoples' feelings or the vibe of the entire room. They have to deal both with their own negative emotions and those of others.

Imagine this scenario: Your spouse has been stressed out by an incident at work. They get home and are exhausted. Soon after, despite having a good day in general, you start feeling stressed due to the energy they are releasing.

HSP's natural tendency to pick up the emotional states of others can be a constant source for conflict. It can be difficult to recognize what you're feeling, and why. Are you worried about your job interview? Is it the interviewer seeming distracted? Or is there something else? How about the "rude encounter" on the route to the interview. Maybe the coffee shop worker was just having a bad day, and didn't realize that he was exclaiming it in his body language.

Yes, everyone experiences inner conflict in some way. But for highly sensitive people, the daily struggle of absorbing emotions from others is an everyday struggle. Some people can feel guilty for harboring anger, sadness or anxiety. Sometimes, though they are clearly theirs, they feel so overwhelmed by them that it is hard for them to overcome. You don't need to be a HSP to control your emotional reactions. To get out of your "rut", you must take a step back to allow your feelings and thoughts to be processed in a more helpful manner. You must learn self-regulation skills.

Chapter 11: Understanding and managing negative emotions

If you are an anxious, sensitive person, then you understand how vital it is that you learn healthy ways of managing your emotions. Here are some of the best techniques for dealing with and getting over negative feelings.

1. Allow yourself to be present and allow your emotions to guide you for a while.

It seems that highly sensitive people have difficulty accepting the idea their emotions may be incorrect. The emotion is a reflection of a failure in one's ability to fulfill one's promises. They then try to suppress it.

This is why it's best to accept emotions as normal parts of human behavior. You may feel angry, but you would prefer to be feeling something else than irritation. It is normal to feel angry. But, it's okay to feel agitated right now. Pushing the issue away will only prolong the situation. It will still exist if you continue to oppose it.

It is important that you don't feel hurt or anxious when you are feeling unwell. But, you need to first feel those emotions to be able fully to let go.

This can be as simple as sitting in silence, wrapped in a blanket, and working on the problem. For truly unblocking an emotion and processing it, journaling, confiding with trusted friends, and sometimes crying out loud can be helpful. Crying can be nature's natural way to express how you feel. It helps to reduce pain, detoxify and cleanse the body. You may even yell, hit a pillow, tear up paper, depending on whether or not you are in a safe space. All these actions help to get out of a rut and move the feelings forward.

2. Do not be embarrassed by the feelings that may arise.

I've seen many HSPs having a lot trouble with this. HSPs are more sensitive than others and have higher levels of perfectionionism. They may feel an unpleasing emotion. This is a sign of their flaws. Also, being flawed means that they are not worthy of affection. For a better response, treat yourself like a friend. Do you think your loved ones will be less affectionate if they are experiencing pain? Most likely, not. The same principle applies to conversations with oneself. It is important to be open to the emotions that result from any situation. Refusing to accept your emotions is not a way to manage them. Acceptance in the present is crucial.

3. Negative emotional triggers should be avoided

What doesn't work when dealing with negative emotions? Doom and gloom. It doesn't really matter where it originated or who sent the message. Any negative influence on your ability to recover from adverse emotions can be detrimental. You must avoid stressful situations when you are dealing with unhappiness.

It's almost always negative so avoid watching the news. Turn your attention away form those who are constantly looking for reasons to be unhappy or are obsessed with negative thoughts. Reflect on your relationship with the people in you life and what it feels like to spend time with them. If you feel more negative after spending time with someone, you might need to adjust your relationship with them. There are people that are just too difficult to deal with, like your mother or coworker. It's time to set boundaries. We will discuss this in a later chapter.

4. Take care to take good care of yourself and your body.

HSPs tend to feel more negative emotions if they aren't well rested, tired, or stressed. Emotions can seem to consume you, but they are a part your body. Even though it is a feeling, they can have physical effects such as an increase cortisol or an increase your heart rate. This is why it is so important to take care your physical health.

Healthy living is as easy as it sounds. Eating regularly, eating healthy foods, exercising, getting enough sleep, and getting enough rest are all key factors to your good health. These are the foundations of good health and wellness. Increased physical activity can help with weight loss, as well as increasing endorphin levels. It also protects your body against the dangers of stress. For highly sensitive people, it is important to be able "clear away" negative emotions and process ones experiences. They may require more sleep than the average person.

5. Accept that emotions may be temporary.

These intense feelings can make it seem impossible to control. A bad mood can also make it difficult to see other people around you. This only makes matters worse. If they aren't buckle under the pressure it is because they are less capable than you. This isn't true. Everyone has their own set of problems. Many people conceal their weaknesses and problems in the same manner as you.

Negative emotions are only temporary. The sensation of falling into a deep, dark place can make you believe that it will never end. This is a very emotional feeling that you don't understand on an intellectual level.

Unsatisfaction with your partner can cause a ripple effect in your view of your relationship. Do you think things will go on as they are? You may think you should leave the situation before it is too late. The feeling quickly fades. The intensity of the feeling begins to diminish. The intensity gradually fades away and life returns to normal. It is important to remember that these feelings, while normal, are only temporary.

6. Avoid thinking in black and white.

It's easy to get caught up in negative emotions when they seem overwhelming. It's like we must face the world alone, or our problem will overcome us regardless of how hard we try. This is what's known as "black & white thinking," which refers to the tendency of thinking in extremes. You can be either a spectacular success or a complete failure. It's a mental stumblingblock that can increase bad feelings. If you use terms like "always" or "never," you could find yourself stuck in an all-or none mindset. Sometimes the truth lies somewhere between.

You don't have to choose between two solutions. There are always other options. Consider all possible solutions, starting with the first three. You cannot anticipate what will happen in every situation, so you should let go. Think about what you have control over. What can I do for others? This is the time when you feel empowered and start to see a path forward.

7. Take the time to reconnect with your body so you can step out of your head.

If you are anxious, speed up your breathing. It's often better to first accelerate when your heart and mind race than to force everything to slow down. A quick stroll around the block is a good idea. If you want to do push-ups, or a jog, then this is the place for you. Any movement that gets you moving will work. Movement helps in the release of adrenaline. The process can be slowed down gradually once your body is in tune with your mental state. Are you unable to do strenuous movements? Try power poses. You can also influence your mental health and well-being by the way you sit.

To help you relax, you can also use your body's sensations to bring you back to normal. Deep breathing exercises and yoga are some of the best relaxation methods.

Hot showers are also very effective, as they are both relaxing and cleansing. You can even use visualization for your advantage. You can even visualize yourself taking a hot shower to remove negative energy and bring in more positive energy.

Look at the physical sensations or rituals that make you feel calmer and more centered. As soon as you begin using the habits, you will see a difference in your body's ability to detect the physical cue for healing. This will lead to a dramatic improvement in your overall health.

8. Find a creative way to express your creativity.

Everyone needs to express themselves creatively. There's something for everybody, no matter what your interests are, such as writing, painting, singing, needlework, and even music. Highly sensitive people can best manage difficult emotions by having a way through which they can express themselves.

To redirect your intense feelings of being sensitive to your environment, it's best to use that awareness to create something constructive. It shouldn't surprise you that many of the most amazing works of art are born out of difficult events or terrible experiences.

9. Be supportive of your body's natural rhythms.

HSPs thrive when they have regular outlets to recharge. They thrive on a fixed schedule. Make your bedroom a peaceful haven where you can unwind at night. This will make it easier to sleep well and get restful sleep. If you want to avoid seasonal affective disorder (also called SAD), make sure that your bedroom is well-lit in the mornings. You should make an effort to maintain a tidy workplace. You can feel more relaxed when you are faced with difficult situations by having lavender essential oils available. A set of earphones is a must to enable you to listen or meditate.

You can be proactive and ensure your environment supports you.

10. Maintain a healthy blood sugar level.

If you are feeling irritable and foggyheaded, it is time to examine your hunger levels. It is best not to have difficult conversations with hungry people. It will not result in a positive outcome. This conversation should not be difficult unless it is about "where do we eat?"

Also, reduce the intake of stimulants. Many HSPs hate sugar and caffeine because they are more sensitive. You can start to pay more attention to how your body reacts when you consume these chemicals.

11. Establish a mindfulness-based routine that you can continue to practice.

It could be a form meditation or yoga. The goal is to establish a practice that will allow you to observe your thoughts distantly. If your emotions get triggered, it is like they are taking you over. The feeling of being swept along by the current of your thoughts is like a river. It's like standing on a bank watching the current of thoughts.

Mindful breathing activates the parasympathetic nervous network, which aids in sleep, digestion and other functions. To create a little bubble, simply inhale into your nose and exhale out through your mouth. Also, square breathing and diaphragmatic breathing are beneficial.

Instead of suppressing the nervous system in stressful situations, try grounding. It allows your nervous to return to normal and can help you relax. You can ground yourself by simply focusing your attention on your breathing.

Highly sensitive people tend to be more susceptible to negative emotions. This side effect is not something you should be aware of, however self-aware you may be. HSPs often feel that the emotion will last forever when it gets strong. Those low moments are part of your life. They are just the same as highs and as valuable, if they are not already. They are unpleasant, and if they are not dealt with, they can become a trap.

Negative emotions are meant to make you feel more balanced, to teach and to remind you of the blessings in your life. You don't have the right to remain in negative emotions forever.

Be confident in your abilities to affect your environment, alter the situation, or overcome any challenges. You can stop life spinning out of control. You all have the power to change your own lives. We can have an influence on their development and emotions, but we cannot change them.

Chapter 12: How to Deal With Overstimulation

Infancy is when we learn how to regulate our emotions by our interactions and with our parents. These abilities can be used by adults on a regular basis, without our conscious thought. As we have already mentioned, "emotional regulation" is the ability to adjust and control one's feelings, particularly when they can be severe or unfavorable. It is important to not "feel better" or stop feeling. However, we need to learn how to manage our emotions and feelings so that we are not powerless. Deficiency can cause long-term psychological problems.

It's likely that you were highly sensitive as children and are now highly sensitive. Most likely, your parents tried their best to comfort you and calm you down when you wept as children. You might also find them whispering or humming softly to comfort you. This helped you feel better and allowed you to release stress. We can strengthen and develop our ability control and regulate emotions through conscious application of similar techniques in adulthood.

If you feel overwhelmed by emotions, it is best to control them. You would not have sobbed if your parents shouted at you, reprimanded or kept you locked in a room all by yourself as a child. It is important to learn how to control your emotions and not allow yourself to get too upset in stressful situations. This will increase your tension and cause irritation. It won't help you calm down.

While it's true that you can be overwhelmed with emotion and overstimulated to the point of feeling the need to flee, there are methods to help you reduce stress levels and quickly regain control. These are tried-and true methods to help you recover if you feel overwhelmed by overstimulation.

Find silence.

A quiet place you love is your home, the library and a bookshop. Cafes are wonderful, however, they can be quite noisy. It is important that you remember that quiet spaces may not always be within your home. However, it is possible to find quiet places in isolated parks or lakes.

Participate in familiar music.

Play a song you're familiar with from your own playlist and get close to it. Even though new sensory input may be difficult for some, familiar sounds can often be soothing.

Place your phone in airplane mode or turn off.

These are great alternatives to using your phone. You might find it very useful to avoid distractions such as television and radio when you use this strategy.

You can concentrate on the present by closing all your eyes.

Sensory overload sufferers will cover their ears and close their eyes as a matter instinct. If you are experiencing extreme reactions, these precautions might help to prevent them. Surprisingly closing your eyes can sometimes be helpful in dealing with excessive sound. The brain isn't aware of this distinction, and it only has large amounts of sensory information to process.

You can indulge in artistic creations.

Seek out something beautiful and let your mind wander. This category could also include literature, artwork, music or street art. You should be inspired by what you see. There is a tremendous amount of energy to be gained.

Politely request silence.

Many HSPs avoid this tactic because they want to be helpful to others. Although it's not suitable for every environment (e.g. construction sites), you can tell your roommate or coworkers what you need if they are constantly talking or listening to loud music.

It's safe to say, "I've been experiencing a really tough period and am feeling overwhelmed." You are okay with being quiet for a few minutes?

It is best to leave the situation as soon as you can.

Take control of your emotions and avoid situations that cause you to feel stressed. The ideal solution to stress is to get out of an office. But, if the place you're stuck in is noisy, packed, or crowded, it's best to just leave the space. If you find yourself outside, and it's busy, find somewhere quiet to sit. If you have a limited time or are looking for solitude, a single bathroom is a good option.

Use the box breathing method to your benefit.

If you find yourself stuck in a stressful environment, deep breathing exercises can be your best friend. Box breathing can be used when you feel anxious or stressed because it is easy to remember.

After you have counted to 4, take a slow inhale from your nose. Keep it going. Take a slow, steady inhale through the mouth after you've counted four more times. You can continue this for up to four minutes.

Use the box breathing technique to calm yourself so that it is easier to use when you're stressed.

Go outside for some fresh air.

You can find a sense of calm when you take a walk in the park or hike up a favorite route. It can be very peaceful and refreshing to go back to nature when all the noise of modern life is too much. Many studies have demonstrated that exposure to sunlight can boost energy and mood. Walking in the quiet streets or through an office park is another option.

Spend some time studying.

A little bit if healthy escapism is good to the soul. And there's nothing like a good read to help you get lost in another world. The best way to unwind is through books. University of Sussex found subjects who read for just six minutes had lower heart beats, less muscle tension, higher stress levels, and had lower heart rates than those who didn't read.

Take a break from the stressors that make you feel stressed by reading a relaxing book in your own quiet space. Enjoy a cup with hot chocolate, tea, or coffee to increase your relaxation.

Pay attention to how you look.

Self-care can be defined as activities that provide relief or revitalization. But, taking care to your body is the best way to self-care. To rejuvenate your senses, pay attention to your body.

You can take a long and hot bath.

You can de-stress faster and more effectively by taking a hot tub or shower if your stress levels are high. Warm water helps release serotonin, which is a neurotransmitter that aids in stress relief. A neurotransmitter called serotonin, it regulates mood, appetite, sleep, and social functioning. Baths can be a great way to unwind and also provide aromatherapy benefits. Even more relaxation can be achieved by mixing lavender, rose and chamomile essential oil with other relaxing ingredients.

Refrain from using social networks.

If you feel overwhelmed and overstimulated it is important to not engage in any activities that may further aggravate your symptoms. While we enjoy social media, they can be irritating and even annoying over time. Due to our deep differences on so many topics, we have turned to social media for expression.

A large number of social media users are open to supporting political and social content. No matter your political views or socioeconomic status, there will be something that angers you or saddens. Avoid using social media to make you feel worse.

Chapter 13: Deep vs. shallow breath

Even though it seems simple, breathing can be a crucial part of being more present. By paying attention to how we breathe, we can become more present in the moment and more focused. Most people only inhale through their mouth and nose, so they breathe less deeply than they should. Deep breathing can activate abdominal muscles. This is often referred to as "belly breath". When you are feeling anxious or worried, taking quick deep breaths can be a natural reaction. Deep breathing allows our brains to signal that everything is fine and allows us to relax our bodies as well as our minds.

If you find yourself taking deep breaths, or just skipping them all together, either close your eyes. To determine if you are breathing deep or shallowly, hold your hands against your stomach and chest. Slowly inhale. Your breathing will be shallower & faster if you only move your chest.

To practice belly breath, inhale deeply through your nose. Think of air traveling from your nose through your nostrils, up your neck, past the lungs, to the lower half of your abdomen, as you inhale and exhale through mouth. When you first try this, your chest may feel tight or restricted. Take a deep, slow inhale and breathe out through the nose. Keep inhaling for as long and as necessary to remove all air from your stomach. If you are trying to relax through your breathing, the exhale will be important.

Swallowing activates the sympathetic nerve system, the area of the brain that controls fight-or-flight reactions. Inhaling activates a portion of our neural system which is only activated while the body's at rest. You will be taken completely by surprise when you take a deep, inhale deeply and exhale. Exhaling and exhaling the same way as before communicates your state of relaxation to the brain and body.

The predisposition to be overstimulated can't be completely avoided. Every one of these situations has the potential of becoming overstimulating because of the processing of multiple stimuli. Exposed people cannot be avoided as this would result in boring, controlled lives.

Sometimes it is necessary for you to take short periods of overstimulation to be able to lead an active lifestyle and to learn new things, take risks, follow your life goals and take chances. Although overstimulation can be uncomfortable, it is only dangerous to your health to continue being exposed for a prolonged period of time, without giving your nervous systems a break. In order to reduce their sensitiveness, highly sensitive individuals should practice relaxation.

Do you remember feeling guilty because you couldn't help someone in crisis or when you had to decline a request from someone? Being forced to socialize with your coworkers and driving a family member to the airport at night after work is over is a sign of stress. Due to guilt and obligation you may have said "yes" despite your internal voice telling you otherwise.

Being an HSP may make it more difficult to take good care of yourself and to set healthy boundaries. High-sensitive people face the greatest challenges when it comes to dealing with stress and guilt. If you don't want to disappoint someone, it is better to hurt their feelings. This is why you may sacrifice your own wants and needs in order help them.

The guilt intensity dial is higher for highly sensitive individuals than it is for the other 80%. HSPs can become more distressed when others are upset. HSPs are more likely to try to help someone else even if their own tanks are empty. They may be able to save someone's lives or offer a way to feel better. Highly sensitive people tend to be more open to helping others than they are to dealing with the emotions of distress or the frustrations caused by their energetic limitations.

The feeling of guilt can be multifaceted. It can cause a host of emotions including regret, worry, grief, shame, and self-doubt. HSPs will want to avoid the unpleasant feelings of guilt for as long and as possible. However, this will only work in the short-term. The long-term consequences of making these sacrifices include anger, sadness, anxiety, and resentment.

Shame and guilt can be socially accepted emotions. It is impossible to feel it if you don't have people around. Shame seems designed to keep us in our social circle, and punish us for minor violations. We, as humans, used groups to survive. If we were persistently bad behaved, we would be kicked off the group.

You are less guilty if you believe you did something wrong than you would be if you believed you were innocent. Even if the guilt does not hold true, it is still a possibility.

Is Guilt Real Always?

Guilt can be seen as a type of debt. Many people mistakenly believe it can be paid by suffering. We believe that guilt can be repaid if we continue to complete certain actions.

On the other hand, emotions don't work like this. If you don't process them correctly, they'll sit in the digestive tract like a giant, fatty lump. It is wrong to believe guilt is always justified. Some people are truly toxic. They have an unusual but powerful gift of making others feel guilty for things they believe are vital to their survival. Are you one of these people? They seem to sow seeds in your mind of guilt with every word you speak.

Do some research before giving in to your guilt. How many of them have you ever had contact with? And how long have they been with you? Does it seem possible that they could be partially to blame? It is futile to attempt to pay your debts if it does not work. There is no debt you owe.

However strong that feeling of guilt seems, it's a false flag. You don't have to feel guilty. Fake guilt acts like fake currency. It circulates regardless of how hard you try to eliminate it. It is illegal and must be destroyed.

HSP Shame:

HSPs are known for having a greater tolerance for shame than other individuals. They feel emotions more strongly than others. However, their awareness of these emotions is part of the reason. Their increased sensitivity allows them to use strategies such as being mindful and cautious before deciding to act. They avoid shame and hide anything that could make them dislike others. They are also considerate and do their best to avoid causing harm and are able to anticipate the long-term implications of their actions. They have an inborn ability to recognize shame, and resist impulses that may lead to it.

Poor parenting and punishments such as shaming are more likely to affect HSPs. They can also feel shame for being neglected, abandoned, or ignored. Even though it may not make sense, it encourages them to work harder in order for them to receive the love they desire.

Most people are quick to blame others for what they did not do. Or minimize their responsibility with statements like "I don't really mean it," or "that wasn't really part my job." Sometimes they may give the impression they are not afraid of what they did by saying "This doesn't apply to me--I am above all that" or "I don't care what people think about me." Sometimes, they make others feel inferior. These coping mechanisms can be used by people with high sensitive personalities, but they don't seem to use as many because they avoid embarrassing behaviour. They adjust to the preferences of others. Their goal is to be perfect, error-free and extraordinarily generous. They achieve more than what they think they can. Nobody can accuse them that they haven't tried or achieved anything.

However, sometimes this obsession with detail can lead one to severely limit their life. Since shame is not a cause of shame, it's hard to tell when you aren't feeling shame. We're not being spontaneous, warm or loving. We aren't reaching out for what we want or thinking about what made our lives happy. We don't need to be ashamed of our actions until we make that realization.

Many people remember being humiliated as children. For some, it was when they were potty-trained, when they were punished for staying in the room, or when someone spanked them for something they weren't. This realization was especially distressing for people who realized their differences from the majority was unacceptable. Either our sensitivity or the reactions of others made us feel shame. If a parent reacts harshly, for example, children caught stealing can feel shame. Children who are particularly sensitive, however, may feel more guilt.

It is acceptable to accept that the moment at which one officially joins the human race is the moment in which they experience shame. This is similar to experiencing shame's awful anguish for the first time. This will cause you to try harder to avoid suffering it again.

It is important to remember that shame is closely linked with your HSP characteristics. This is because you are empathic as well as compassionate. These are essential qualities for relationships as well as being a loved friend, parent, relative, and partner. It shows you care about other people and their well-being that you feel guilty. It is something that we can strive for. But healthy boundaries, self-care and self-care are important, which we will discuss in a separate section.

It takes a lot to get over shame. Fortifying yourself is the most important thing. It is essential to feel loved and confident about yourself.

Even if guilt cannot be eliminated completely, it can be reduced and transformed into self-acceptance. It's all about listening to your inner voice and being willing put yourself first over other people.

Instead of doing what is expected of you, consider what it would be like to do. You may appear to be sacrificing a basic need when you lower your boundaries in order care for another person. You can avoid anger or estrangement by acting only in your self-interest.

If you are deciding whether or no to a request, think about your availability to assist. Your friends should only accept your "yes" when you are ready.

Before you care for someone else, it is essential to determine your needs. By practicing self-compassion, you can free yourself from the pressures of perfectionism and duty. You can also turn your empathy inward. You can say the following to yourself:

"I'm trying to do my best with the resources I have."

"Please allow me the grace to be gentle with you."

"I want myself to be exactly who I am"

Two of your most sensitive talents as an HSP are your ability to empathize. These skills are what make you a good friend, parent or partner. It is an indication that you are compassionate and interested in others' well-being that you feel guilty when you do. Although this is not necessarily a bad thing it can be controlled with self-care and good limits.

Our emotional and empathy abilities make us feel guilty for not answering "yes" or offering assistance to others. It may seem like a great idea to sacrifice your own needs in order not to feel guilty in the short-term, but this will only lead you to resentment anger, anxiety, depression, and unhappiness later on. If you can learn to prioritize your needs and practice self-compassion, shame will be transformed into self-acceptance. In this way, you can be who you really are and interact with people in a real way.

Chapter 14: Enhancing Self-Esteem

Most people care less about their self-esteem and more about how it affects their day-today lives. HSPs have a tendency to treat self-confidence as if it were clothing that everyone could see. Follow these steps to make a positive impact in your daily life.

Accept thoughts and feelings as they are.

You shouldn't judge them. They are temporary and easily changed. They are a result of the mind and body.

Don't depend on others to make sure you feel valued.

You will undoubtedly fall prey to another person. You must become the sole bearer of your power. You can't be a label, position or affiliation that gives you value. These are not relevant information. It is vital that you maintain your self-esteem when someone or something happens in your life.

You should embrace your thinking outside the box.

HSPs can be called among the most gifted artists on the planet. Why? Why? Because they have a curiosity and are open to asking questions about the status quo. HSPs are different from those who fear to dream big, and they can achieve their goals.

Utilize your emotional intelligence.

HSPs can pick up subtleties and details that others may miss, and they can hear what is being said without having to be told. It might surprise you to find out that highly sensitive people are able to communicate with others, listen, empathize, and be great marketers.

Allow others to leave feedback easily.

Even though they are excellent communicators most sensitive people have trouble catching their breath during presentations or meetings. The same goes for people who are sensitive to harsh statements. This can cause them to be uncomfortable for several days or even weeks. If you are a HSP, be ready for high-stakes conversations ahead of being questioned. Make a list of common work questions to be answered in your response bank.

"Permit to return to me."

"That is a very good question. What are your thoughts?

"Thank you so much for your input. Give me some time for my thoughts to process what you just said.

Don't react. Instead, respond.

It is crucial to have resilience and high functioning personality in the face the unexpected. By practicing mindfulness techniques, you can discern the difference between your emotional reaction (or trigger event) and your mental health. You should not let anxiety control your life. Stress is more prominent in high-functioning people because they have a tendency to experience more intense feelings.

It's not a good idea, or even a good idea, to get angry at your partner for leaving dirty dishes in his sink. It is a good idea to take a deep, slow breath and count up to five before you react in stressful situations. This will allow you to regain control of how your impulses are responding.

You can ask for a timeout if your words are something you regret or that you realize you did not mean. Before reacting, it is a good idea to make a list. It is fine to break off a relationship before moving on. It shows maturity, critical thinking, and self-control. These are all qualities you should be proud to display.

Chapter 15: Was it your belief that this would work?

Why would I go the extra mile to help you

What would you describe yourself as?

On the plus side they often achieve their goals. These people are able to set boundaries and they don't have any problems. Neglecting the needs of others and demeaning them can only lead to more problems in relationships.

It's worth noting that few highly sensitive people communicate aggressively. HSPs are attracted to people who share their values.

Passive: This is the opposite of an aggressive communicator. They will put the needs of others before their own. Even if this means that they may have to sacrifice their own needs. They tend to appear ambiguous and unclear. This type of communication is how the "yes" man or women came to be. Here are some examples.

"I cannot decide...what do YOU think?"

"Yes, I can manage that for you,"

"It is not my area but I believe I can help."

It is easy to build relationships with others in this group. Who wouldn't want someone to respond quickly to their needs and wants? Inauthenticity, however, can reduce the importance of those relationships. If they say no, their 'yeses are meaningless.

Passive aggressive: These people dress up as sheep and are wolves. They promise to do whatever it takes to make you happy, but then don't. They might insult you, but it is done passively and with passive language. Alternately, you can use nonverbal aggressive. These people don't speak their emotions but are in a state of anger. This type communicator may do any of these:

You can pretend that they are "fine" even though their tone might suggest otherwise

Be malicious or spiteful in a nonaggressive fashion

Don't be afraid to sulk and not explain your needs

These people are often a mixture of personalities. Despite the fact that they don't always follow through on their promises, they appear kind and helpful. They will only avoid conflict and satisfy one's needs but they won't go far enough for healthy communication or personal growth.

It is the communication style everyone seeks. Being assertive means that you can find ways to balance the needs and wants of others while still maintaining your own goals. They communicate what they mean and don't hesitate to say so. It is their duty to advocate for themselves. However, they are respectful of the opinions of others.

Statements like these are in action

"I am having difficulties with something. I would like to have a conversation with you. Are you available to meet?

"I wish you could have my assistance, but I have other plans."

"Could your please do me a huge favour? I'm struggling to complete everything. I would appreciate any help you could give me if you had a second.

This group takes care of their own needs, while also considering others. If they are capable of helping and show a willingness to, they will. If they cannot help, they won't claim that they can and then dodge the question. There are no ambiguities about their needs or wants, nor about their ability to meet them.

Assertiveness Techniques

If someone is too sensitive it can be difficult to advocate for their rights in a calm and constructive manner. However, this is not unusual. They may be viewed as a burden by others who speak too much and don't care about their feelings or points of views. HSPs hate aggressive communication due to their vulnerability to hurt. They would rather avoid conflict altogether, in the hopes that it would resolve itself.

HSPs can be difficult to manage and often get stepped on by others. However, this does not stop them from being assertive when necessary. It is possible to learn skills such as managing emotions, setting boundaries and communicating your thoughts. The following strategies will help you to be more assertive.

1. Communicate using assertive writing

I find it very beneficial to communicate my concerns in writing whenever I deal with a conflict. Written communication can not only provide instant cathartic release but also clarifies the situation and is useful for open communication when used correctly.

Writing a letter to someone about a disagreement is important. These statements are crucial because they express your view and emotional needs in a manner that doesn't place blame on the opposing party.

A persuasive letter should be concise and explain the situation clearly. Here is a template that you can use to help get started.

Greetings,

While bringing up this subject (conflict/misunderstanding) is difficult for me, I believe that it is necessary to do so (despite my reluctance). I am writing you this letter because I feel that writing allows for me to express myself better.

Recently, I feel betrayed and abandoned by someone I love (insert situation). When (the event) happens, I get the impression that (whatever my emotional need is not met) am in control.

I have felt my thoughts drawn to this recently and don't want it to go unnoticed any longer. While I would love to see this problem resolved quickly, I don't want to ignore how I feel.

Sincerely,

You

2. You must be aware of how people perceive you.

People's movements and words can reveal much about them. Some people may see the humility of HSPs as weakness. They might attempt to profit from them by seeing their modesty as weakness. You should avoid certain words and phrases that can make you seem assertive. Here are some examples.

Avoid using the word "just." It reduces the impact of a statement if you use the term "just" because it makes you appear defensive.

"I'm not" statements. People will often use phrases like "I'm certainly not an expert but ..." to try to sound less aggressive or arrogant. But, it can damage the validity of their message.

"I can't..." statements. A statement that begins with "I don't '...'"" implies that you have lost control by using passive phrasing.

Answering with question. It is less important to answer with a question than it is to simply state an idea.

Apologies. If you say "I am sorry for any inconvenience caused to you," it is an indication that you are apologizing. You come across as untrustworthy.

Too emphatic punctuation. Consider the following text reply: "Thanks for your help!" ; " This example shows that your use of emoticons or exclamation points in written or SMS messages is self-conscious.

You should also remember that body language like hunched shoulders, folded arms and no eye contact can communicate defensiveness and lackluster confidence. Speaking in front of crowds is a great way for you to improve your body language. A public speaking club is a great way to increase your confidence and show off your stage presence.

3. Take nothing too personally.

When people can't deal with their own problems, it is easy to transfer their negativity onto their friends. This realization will help you create a filter that is more sensitive to other people's feelings. It is important that you understand why you react defensively in certain situations. This will help you recognize that certain people have more power over you than necessary. You are the only one who can make you feel inferior.

4. Take control of you happiness and well being.

It's important that you realize that your happiness doesn't depend on other people's happiness. Many HSPs find themselves unhappy because they care too deeply about what other people think, need their approval, or don't take enough time to let go and enjoy the moment.

5. Consider yourself equal to other people.

HSPs might feel inferior to other HSPs, which can impact their work and personal relationships.

It is vital to realize that even people who don't have them, others may also be insecure. While everyone faces the same challenges in life, our attitudes towards life and how we relate to others affects how we treat the world around and ourselves. Instead of focusing on what others think, try focusing on how you perceive yourself.

6. Give yourself time to process your responses.

Instead of saying only what you think people want, say what they actually need to hear. HSPs may be in a difficult place when it comes honesty.

Do you feel like not going out for dinner tonight. Talk to your friend. Before you say anything that is positive and will be welcomed by others, take your own time. Ask yourself, "Is it really what you want to say or do?" Before answering.